Immunopharmacology
Strategies for Immunotherapy

Immunopharmacology
Strategies for Immunotherapy

Editor
Shakti N. Upadhyay

CRC Press
Boca Raton London New York Washington, D.C.

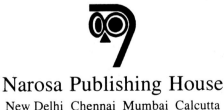

Narosa Publishing House
New Delhi Chennai Mumbai Calcutta

Shakti N. Upadhyay
National Institute of Immunology
New Delhi 110016, India

Library of Congress Cataloging-in-Publication Data:

A catalog record for this book is available from the Library of Congress.

Exclusive distribution in North America only by CRC Press LLC

Direct all inquiries to CRC Press LLC, 2000 N.W. Corporate Blvd., Boca Raton,
Florida 33431. Email: orders@crcpress.com

No claim to original U.S. Government works
International Standard Book Number 0-8493-0951-4
Printed in India

Preface

The consequences of diseases involving the immune system now appear to have much wider impact on health care and management. Although over the last decade our understanding of the basic immunological mechanisms underlying various diseases has increased considerably, the applications of these research findings for drug development have not been fully exploited. This book attempts to bring together contributions from experts involved with different aspects of immunology including topics ranging from immunological interactions and responses, effector mechanisms and targets for the modulation of immune response, with a view to analyzing the current strategies for immunotherapy and exploring the new immunopharmacological approaches for prevention and treatment of diseases by manipulating the immune system. We hope that the information presented in this book would be of interest to the researchers and will stimulate new ideas for further scientific investigations.

SHAKTI N UPADHYAY

Acknowledgements

We acknowledge the following for sponsoring the Indo-French Symposium on Immunopharmacology, held at the National Institute of Immunology, New Delhi, on the occasion of the Golden Jubilee of India's Independence.

Embassy of France, New Delhi

Pasteur-Merieux-Connaught, India

INSERM, France

National Institute of Immunology, New Delhi

Department of Biotechnology, Government of India

Dabur Research Foundation, Ghaziabad

We especially thank **CEDUST, Embassy of France, New Delhi,** and **Pasteur-Merieux-Connaught, New Delhi,** for providing financial support to publish this volume.

Contents

Immunopharmacology
Strategies for Immunotherapy

Immunopharmacology: Strategies for immunotherapy
S.N. Upadhyay (Ed)

1. Neutralization of IgG Autoantibodies of Autoimmune Patients by Pooled Normal Human Polyspecific IgM: Implication in immunotherapy

**S. Kaveri, T. Vassilev, E. Bonnin, V. Hurez,
A. Pashov, S. Lacroix-Desmazes,
B. Bellon* and M.D. Kazatchkine**
*INSERM U430, Hôpital Broussais, Paris, France

Natural autoantibodies of both the IgM and IgG isotypes reactive with a wide spectrum of membrane-associated, intracellular, nuclear and circulating self antigens, including idiotypes of immunoglobulins, are present in normal serum [1–3]. Most of the NAA characterised so far are polyreactive in that the antibodies are capable of recognizing several self and 'foreign' antigens [2]. Depending on their specificity, natural IgG autoantibodies which have been affinity-purified from human serum exhibit similar or higher degrees of polyreactivity as compared with autoantibodies from patients with autoimmune diseases [4]. Experiments using site-directed mutagenesis have indicated that the complementarity determining region (CDR) 3 in the V_H domain is primarily involved in determining the relative polyreactivity of NAA [5, 6]. Analysis of V genes of natural, of 'foreign antigen'-induced and of autoimmune disease associated human monoclonal antibodies has delineated some of the structural features of the respective antigen-binding sites. Most NAA are directly encoded by germline V genes and are subjected to practically no mutation. In contrast, germline-encoded reactivity to 'foreign antigen' is rare. Several functions have been proposed for NAA under physiological conditions (Box 2). It has been proposed that NAA function primarily to control autoreactivity and immune homeostasis, in healthy individuals. Of essential relevance for autoimmunity, is the role of NAA in participating in the selection of autoreactive B cells and in preventing the uncontrolled expansion of specific autoreactive clones, as well as the ability of NAA through V region-dependent complementary interactions to control autoreactivity in serum under physiological conditions.

A Therapeutic Role for Natural IgG Autoantibodies
Initially used as substitutive therapy in primary and secondary immune deficiencies, pooled normal human polyspecific IgG (IVIg) is increasingly being used in the treatment of autoimmune dieseases [7, 8]. Several mutually non-exclusive mechanisms account for the immunomodulatory properties of IVIg, including the ability of IVIg to neutralize circulating autoantibodies, to inhibit the function of Fc receptors, to modulate cytokine production and complement activation, to regulate the functions and select the repertoires of B and T lymphocytes [9–12].

Therapeutic Potential of Natural IgM Autoantibodies
Serum IgM has been shown to play an important role in controlling the expression of IgG autoreactivity [3, 13]. Thus, under physiological conditions, autoreactive IgG autoantibodies, although present, are hardly detectable in whole serum of a healthy individual, whereas high levels of autoreactivity expressed by IgG become apparent when IgG is isolated from serum prior to being tested for autoantibody activity [3, 13–16]. The addition of purified IgM to autologous IgG suppresses IgG-associated autoreactivity [3]. Regulation of IgG antibody activity by autologous IgM is preferentially operative in controlling reactivity with self antigens more than it is efficient in the case of antibody reactivities against foreign proteins [3]. IgM-dependent regulation of IgG autoreactivity in serum is defective in autoimmune conditions, such as autoimmune thyroiditis and SLE [3, 16]. In addition, loss of detectable IgG autoantibody activity in the serum of patients in remission of ANCA-positive vasculitis was shown to be associated with the generation of IgM anti-idiotypes directed against the patient's acute phase IgG autoantibodies, indicating that IgM may suppress pathogenic autoantibodies of the IgG isotype in remission of autoimmune disease [17, 18]. Testing the reactivity of IgM produced by several EBV-transformed B cell lines has revaled a high degree of connectivity between normal IgM and variable regions of IgG autoantibodies [19]. Variable region-dependent connectivity between immunoglobulins, e.g. between IgG and autologous IgM or between IgG molecules within the IgG fraction of the serum of an individual, contribute to immune networks and to the maintainance of the homeostasis of autoreactivity under physiological conditions [2, 20]. Infusion of relatively small amounts of homologous natural IgM antibodies prevent the development of diabetes in the IDDM model of the NOD mouse [21]. The deviated pattern of utilization of the VH7183 gene that characterizes the immunoglobulin repertoire of adult NOD mice was also shown to be reversed by neonatal treatment with natural IgM monoclonal antibody [22]. More recently, it has been demonstrated that polyreactive monoclonal IgM antibodies generated from SJL/J mice injected with normal homogenized spinal cord promote central nervous system remyelination when passively transferred into syngeneic mice chronically infected with Theiler's virus induced autoimmune murine encephalomyelitis [23]. Sequence analysis

revealed that these monoclonal antibodies were encoded by identical germline Ig light chain and heavy chain genes with no definitive somatic mutations [23]. An intravenous immunoglobulin preparation enriched in IgM has been shown to be beneficial in post-bone marrow transplantation infections [24] and in patients with sepsis [25]. Further, IgM-enriched preparations of therapeutic immunoglobulins were found to exhibit higher opsonic activity than standard IgG preparations [26]. Together, these observations provide rationale for considering pooled normal IgM obtained from plasma of large mumber of healthy donors for potential therapeutic use in autoimmune diseases, either as supplementary to IVIg or as an alternative to IVIg therapy.

In a recent study, we have demonstrated that pooled normal IgM obtained from plasma of over 2500 healthy donors and processed for potential therapeutic use (IVIgM), suppresses autoantibody activity of IgG purified from the serum of patients [27]. In this overview, we present the lines of evidence which support that the suppression of autoantibody activity by IVIgM is mediated through interactions with idiotypes of autoantibodies.

IVIgM Inhibits Autoantibody Activity of Patients with Autoimmune Disease

We observed that IVIgM dose-dependently inhibited the binding of IgG purified from the serum of patients with SLE, autoimmune thyroiditis, acquired von Willebrand disease, anti-FVIII autoimmune disease and autoimmune uveitis to their respective target autoantigens (Fig. 1). In the case of anti-DNA and anti-TG autoantibodies, IVIgM was shown to block the binding to the self antigens of patients' autoantibodies that had been affinity-purified on Sepharose-bound antigen. No inhibition of autoantibody activity was observed when human monoclonal IgM was used, indication that the inhibitory effect of IVIgM was mediated by variable regions of IgM. IVIgM that was depleted of its rheumatoid factor activity by subjecting it to Fc-Sepharose column strongly inhibited the binding of anti-Tg and anti-DNA autoantibodies to their corresponding target antigens. Furthermore, a human monoclonal IgM rheumatoid factor and IgM purified from sera of patients with rheumatoid arthritis, did not exert any inhibitory activity on autoantibodies tested. These results suggest that the observed blocking effect of the pooled IgM preparation is not related to the presence of rheumatoid factor activity in the preparation.

IVIgM that had been depleted in its content in natural anti-TG autoantibodies by affinity chromatography, inhibited the binding of anti-TG IgG to TG to the same extent as did unfractionated IVIgM. The latter result demonstrating that the inhibitory effect of IVIgM on autoantibody activity was not dependent on its ability to compete with IgG autoantibodies for the binding to the autoantigen but rather on an interaction between variable regions of IgG and IgM. These conclusions were further supported by the finding that $F(ab')_2$ fragments of IgG containing autoantibody activity were selectively retained by IVIgM upon affintiy chromatography.

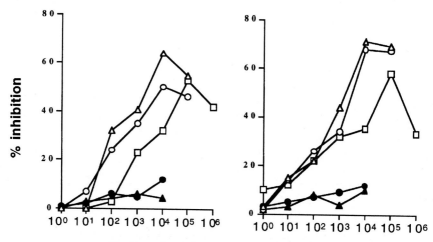

Fig. 1. Inhibition of IgG autoantibody activity by IVIgM. Increasing amounts of IVIgM (open triangles), IVIgM depleted of its rheumatoid factor activity (open circles), IVIg (open squares), a human monoclonal IgM rheumatoid factor (closed circles), or monoclonal IgM (closed triangles), were co-incubated with a fixed amount of ^{125}I-labeled affinity-purified anti-TG or anti-DNA IgG from a patient with Hashimoto's thyroiditis (left panel) and a patient with SLE (right panel), overnight at 4°C. The binding of ^{125}I-IgG to the corresponding antigen was then assessed. Abscissa indicates molar ratios between competitor immunoglobulin and ^{125}I-IgG autoantibody.

Immobilized IVIgM Selectively Retains IgG Autoantibody Activity Upon Affinity Chromatography

F(ab′)$_2$ fragments of IgG isolated from the serum of patients with Hashimoto's thyroiditis and patients with anti-FVIII autoimmune disease were subjected to affinity chromatography on IVIgM-Sepharose and on Waldenstrom IgM-Sepharose. The amount of anitbody in the acid-eluted fraction of the IVIgM-Sepharose column was 0.06% and 0.22% of loaded F(ab′)$_2$ fragments of IgG of the patient with thyroiditis and of the patient with anti-FVIII autoantibodies, respectively. Specific autoantibody activity of acid-eluted F(ab′)$_2$ fragments, as determined by ELISA and expressed as absorbance units/μg was 128 and 17 times higher than that of unchromatographed F(ab′)$_2$ fragments in the case of anti-TG and anti-FVIII autoantibodies, respectively (Table 1). On the contrary, Waldenstrom IgM-Sepharose affinity column retained only negligible amount of F(ab′)$_2$ fragments of IgG autoantibodies. Specific activity of eluted F(ab′)$_2$ fragments from Waldenstrom IgM-Sepharose affinity column was only 1.7 and 0.08 times higher than that of loaded F(ab′)$_2$ fragments in the case of anti-TG and anti-FVIII autoantibodies respectively (Table 1).

IVIgM Contains Anti-idiotypes Directed Against Disease-Associated Autoantibodies

First indirect evidence for the presence of anti-idiotypic antibodies in the

Table 1. Affinity chromatography of F(ab')$_2$ fragments of IgG autoantibodies on IgM coupled to Sepharose*

	Loaded antibodies		Eluted antibodies		Eluted specific activity/loaded specific activity
	Amount (mg)	Specific activity (OD/μg)	Amount (μg)	Specific activity (OD/μg)	
IVIgM-Sepharose					
F(ab')$_2$ of					
Hashimoto IgG	2.4	0.351	1.5	45	128
F(ab')$_2$ of anti-FVIII IgG	1.8	0.120	4.0	2	16.67
Control IgM-Sepharose					
F(ab')$_2$ of					
Hashimoto IgG	0.8	0.403	0.330	0.694	1.72
F(ab')$_2$ of anti-FVIII IgG	0.374	0.170	0.144	0.015	0.08

*F(ab')$_2$ fragments of IgG purified from the serum of a patient with Hashimoto's thyroiditis and a patient with anti-F.VIII autoimmune disease were loaded on IVIgM-Sepharose and on IgM purified from the plasma of a patient with Waldenstrom's macroglobulinemia, coupled to Sepharose, for two hours at room temperature. The columns were eluted at acid pH. The amount of antibody and specific anti-TG and anti-FVIII autoantibody activity were then assessed in the loaded material and in the acid-eluted fractions of the columns.

pooled preparation of IgM came from the finding that IVIgM bind in a dose dependent manner to F(ab')$_2$ fragments of disease-associated IgG autoantibodies from patients with autoimmune conditions (Fig. 2). The possible occurrence

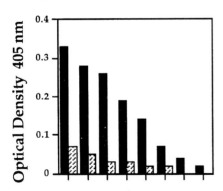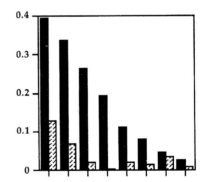

Concentration of IgM (μg/ml)

Fig. 2. Binding of IVIgM of F(ab')$_2$ fragments of disease-associated IgG autoantibodies. Decreasing concentrations of IVIgM (dark bars) or IgM purified from the plasma of a patient with Waldenstrom's macroglobulinemia (hatched bars), were incubated on plates coated with F(ab')$_2$ fragments of IgG of two patients with Hashimoto's thyroiditis (left panels) and F(ab')$_2$ fragments of IgG of two patients with anti-F.VIII autoantibodies.

of anti-idiotypes in a pool of IgM prepared from plasma of large number of healthy donors is further substantiated by the absence of binding of Walsenstrom IgM.

We then demonstrated that IVIgM competitively inhibited the binding of mouse and rabbit anti-idiotypic antibodies to their corresponding idiotypes on anti-TG and anti-FVIII IgG autoantibodies, demonstrating that IVIgM contains anti-idiotypic antibodies directed against the autoantibodies (Fig. 3). Idiotypic interactions provide a basis for the neutralization of circulating autoantibodies and for down-regulation of autoantibody synthesis by pooled normal IgM, as we have previously demonstrated in the case of IVIg [12]. On a molar basis, IVIgM was found to be equivalent to or more efficient than IVIg in its ability to suppress autoantibody activity *in vitro*. The latter finding may relate to the higher extent of polyreactivity of natural IgM antibodies as compared with normal IgG [28].

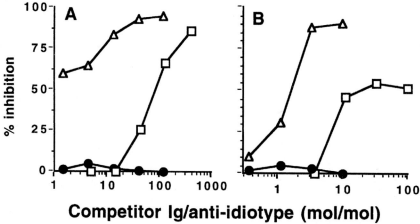

Fig. 3. Competitive binding of IVIgM and heterologous anti-idiotypes to idiotypes of anti-F.VIII and anti-thyroglobulin autoantibodies. Microtiter plates were coated with F(ab')₂ fragments of IgG purified from the plasma of a patient with anti-F. VIII autoimmune disease (left) or with F(ab')₂ fragments of anti-thyroglobulin autoantibodies (right) and incubated with 0.025 μg of anti-idiotypic mAb 20F2 (left panel) or with 0.1 μg of anti-idiotypic monoclonal antibodies 1B4, in the presence of increasing concentrations of IVIgM (open triangles), monoclonal IgM (closed circles) or IVIg (open squares). Bound anti-idiotype was then measured using peroxidase-labeled anti-mouse Ig antibodies. The abscissa represents the molar ratio between competitor immunoglobulin and anti-idiotype.

IVIgM Prevents the Onset of EAU

We further demonstrated immunomodulatory properties of IVIgM *in vivo* using the rat model of EAU. Indeed, as reported for IVIg [29], IVIgM administered at the time of immunization of (LEW × BN) F1 rats with the retinal S antigen, prevented the occurrence of EAU (Table 2). The underlying mechanism in such a protective effect of pooled IgM is currently being investigated.

Table 2. **Effect of infusion of IVIgM on EAU in (LEW × BN) F1 rats**

Treatment	Clinical data		Histological data	
	n positive eyes/total (%)	Score†	*n* positive eyes/total (%)	Score†
None	12/18 (66.7)	2.3 ± 0,2	12/18 (66.7)	4.5 ± 0.3
IVIgM	6/18 (33.3)*	1.7 ± 0.4 NS	6/18 (33.3)*	4,0 ± 0.4 NS
IVIg	0/10 (0)**	0	0/10 (0)**	0

† Score means are calculated from the positive eyes only.
* $p < 0.05$; ** $p < 0.01$, Chi-square test.

Together, these observations indicate for the first time, that pooled normal IgM shares with IVIg the ability to neutralize autoantibody activity through idiotypic interactions. Serum IgM mostly consists of natural germline-encoded autoantibodies, whereas serum IgG also contains significant amounts of immune antibodies to non-self antigens that may not be of direct relevance to network regulation of autoreactivity. Taken together, our observation provide a rationale for considering normal pooled IgM for immunomodulation of autoimmune diesease.

Acknowledgements
This work was supported by Institut National de la Santé et de la Recherche Medicale (INSERM), Centre National de la Recherche Scientifique (CNRS), France, and the Central Laboratory of the Swiss Red Cross (Bern, Switzerland).

References

1. Avrameas, S., Guilbert, B. and Dighiero, G. *Ann. Inst. Pasteur Immunol.* 1981. **132C:** 231.
2. Avrameas, S. *Immunol. Today.* 1991.**12:** 154.
3. Hurez, V., Kaveri, S.V. and Kazatchkine, M.D. *Eur. J. Immunol.* 1993. **23:** 783.
4. Hurez, V., Dietrich, G., Kaveri, S.V. and Kazatchkine, M.D. *Scand J. Immunol.* 1993. **38:** 190.
5. Schettino, E.W., Ichiyoshi,Y. and Casali, P., in Zanetti, M. and Capra, J.D. (Eds.) *The antibodies*, Harwood Academic Publishers, Amsterdam 1996, Vol. **2:** p. 155.
6. Martin, T., Crouzier, R., Weber, J., Kipps, T. and Pasquali, J. *J. Immunol.* 1994. **152:** 5988.
7. Dwyer, J.M.N. *Engl. J. Med.* 1992. **326:** 107.
8. Kazatchkine, M.D. and Morel, A., Eds., *Intravenous Immunoglobulin Research and Therapy* (Parthenon Publishing Group Ltd., London, 1996).
9. Andersson, U.G., Bjork, L., Skansén-Saphir, U. and Andersson, J.P. *Immunol. Rev.* 1994. **139:** 21.
10. Fehr, J., Hofmann, V., and Kappeler, U.N. *Engl. J. Med.*1982. **306:** 1254.
11. Basta, M. and Dalakas, M.C. *J. Clin. Invest.* 1994. **94:** 1729.
12. Kazatchkine, M.D., Dietrich, G., Hurez, V., Ronda, N., Bellon, B., Rossi, F. and Kaveri, S.V. *Immunol. Rev.* 1994. **139:** 79.

13. Adib, M., Ragimbeau, J., Avrameas, S. and Ternynck, T. *J. Immunol.* 1990. **145:** 3807.
14. Berneman, A., Guilbert, B., Eschrich, S. and Avrameas, S. *Mol. Immunol.* 1993. **30:** 1499.
15. Mouthon, L., Nobrega, A., Nicolas, N., Kaveri, S., Barreau, C., Coutinho, A. and Kazatchkine, M. *Proc. Natl. Acad. Sc. USA.* 1995, **92:** 3839.
16. Ronda, N., Haury, M., Nobrega, A., Kaveri, S.V., Coutinho, A. and Kazatchkine, M.D. *Int Immunol.* 1994. **6:** 1651.
17. Rossi, F., Jayne, D.R.W., Lockwood, C.M. and Kazatchkine, M.D. *Clin. Exp. Immunol.* 1991. **83:** 298.
18. Jayne, D.R.W., Esnault, V.L.M. and Lockwood, C.M. *J. Autoimmunity.* 1993. **6:** 207.
19. Rossi, F., Guilbert, B., Tonnelle, C., Ternynck, T., Fumoux, F., Avrameas, S. and Kazatchkine, M.D. *Eur. J. Immunol.* 1990. **20:** 1089.
20. Varela, F. and Coutinho, A. *Immunol. Today.* 1991. **12:** 159.
21. Andersson, A., Forsgren, S., Soderstrom, A. and Holmberg, D. *J. Autoimmunity.* 1991. **4:** 733.
22. Andersson, A., Ekstrand-Hammerstrom, B., Eriksson, B., Overmo, C. and Holmberg, D. *Int.Immunol.* 1994. **6:** 623.
23. Miller, D.J. and Rodriguez, M. *J. Immunol.* 1995. **154:** 2460.
24. Poynton, C.H., Jackson, S., Fegan, C., Barnes, R.A. and Whittaker, J.A. *Bone Marrow Transpl.* 1992. **9:** 451.
25. Haque, K.N., Zaidi, M.H. and Bahakim, H. *Am. J. Dis. Child.* 1988. **142:** 1293.
26. Garbett, N.D., Munro,C.S. and Cole, P.J. *Clin. Exp. Immunol.* 1989. **76:** 8.
27. Hurez, V., Kazatchkine, M.D., Ramanathan, S., Basuyaux, B., Pashov, A., Vassilev, T., De-Kozak,Y., Bellon B. and Kaveri, S.V. *Blood.* 1997. **90:** 4004.
28. Avrameas, S. and Ternynck, T. *Molecular Immunology.* 1993. **30:** 1133.

Immunopharmacology: Strategies for immunotherapy
S.N. Upadhyay (Ed)
Copyright © 1999 Narosa Publishing House, New Delhi, India

2. Chemokine Receptor CCR5 (HIV-1 Coreceptor) Variants Present in India: Selective inactivation of CCR5 and HIV genes by ribozymes

Akhil C. Banerjea

Laboratory of Virology, National Institute of Immunology, New Delhi-110067, India

Abstract

Significant progress has been made in understanding how HIV-1 and HIV-2 make use of chemokine receptors to gain entry into $CD4^+$ and $CD4^-$ host cells. Chemokine receptor CCR5 is used by the virus in the early stages of infection which are predominantly macrophage tropic. During the late stage of infection the virus uses the CXCR-4 (Fusin) which are syncytia inducing T-lymphocyte tropic viruses. These chemokine receptors are 7-transmembrane G-coupled proteins that are involved in signal transduction besides immune regulation. A precise 32 base pair deletion corresponding to the second extracellular loop in the homozygous form was found to afford remarkable protection against repeated exposure to HIV-1 infection (Liu et al., 1996, Huang et al., 1996 Biti et al., 1997, D" Souza et al., 1996, Husain et al., 1998. This deletion results in a frame shift mutation resulting in a severe truncated protein which neither support virus infection nor can participate in signal transduction. This CCR5 gene in the heterozygous form (one wild-type allele and the other Δ32 allele) is found quite frequently (15–20%) among Caucasian people of European heritage but was found remarkably absent (both homo- and heterozygous forms) in large number of Asian and African people in earlier studies. Since genotyping of normal individuals for CCR5 variants could provide important information about the genetic basis of resistance to HIV-1, we screened 100 normal individuals for the Δ32 mutant of CCR5 by amplifying 176 bp region of CCR5 gene by PCR using primers that flanked the deleted region. Only one individual was found to be heterozygous for the Δ32 allele and the rest possessed the wild-type (Wt) CCR5 alleles. We cloned the complete CCR5 gene in a T-tailed vector (pGEM-T-Easy under T7 promoter) and confirmed the precise 32 base pair deletion by sequencing. As expected, the Wt CCR5 only participated in a coreceptor function as measured by CD4-

gp 160 fusion mediated reporter gene (LacZ or Luciferase) activation assay. We have constructed hammer-head ribozyme to selectively inactivate the CCR5 gene and other HIV genes to down regulate the replication of HIV. Chemokine receptors can now be regarded as new attractive targets for antiviral therapies and their study will provide important insights to the understanding of molecular basis of pathogenesis and transmission of HIV.

First Report of the Presence of Δ32 Mutant Allele of CCR5 Gene from Asia

We screened 100 normal healthy individuals from India for the presence of 32 base pair deletion mutant in the CCR5 gene. This was carried out by isolating the genomic DNA from the peripheral blood lymphocytes (Banerjea et al., 1981) and subjecting them to polymerase chain reaction using the primers that flanked the earlier observed 32 base pair deletion. They were.

(1) 5'-Sense-GCGTCTCTCCCAGGAATCATCTTTACC and
(2) Antisense-GATTCCCGAGTAGCAGATGACCATG

This combination of primer pair is expected to amplify 176 bp wild-type CCR5 gene and 144 bp if a 32 base pair deletion is present. The PCR amplified products were analyzed on a 4% agarose gel where a 32 base pair deletion

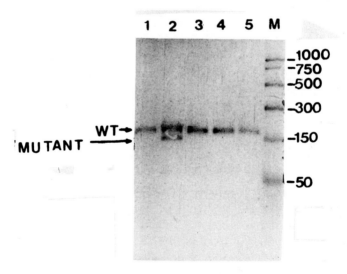

Fig. 1. **CCR5 genotyping of normal unrelated individuals. Genomic DNA from peripheral blood lymphocytes was isolated from normal individuals and subjected to PCR as described before. Amplified products were analyzed on a 4% agarose gel. Wild type CCR5 specific DNA was amplified in all the cases including the control DNA (pCCR5) lane-5. Only one case (sample #5, lane 2) showed the presence of an additional band of about 150 bp size. Lane M represents molecular size of various DNA fragments (PCR markers, Promega Biotech.)**

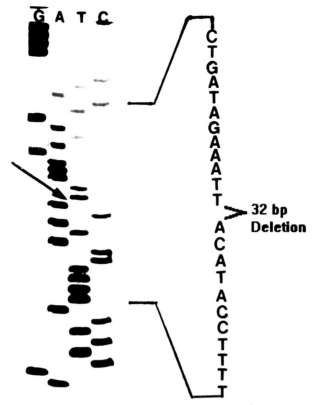

Fig. 2. Sequence analysis of CCR5 mutant clone. The amplified DNA fragments
(176 and ~150 bp from sample #5 were cloned into pGEM-T Easy (Promega
Biotech.) and individual clones were screened for the presence of either 176
or ~150 bp DNA fragment. Purified plasmid DNAs were subjected to *EcoR1*
digestion and analyzed on a 4% agarose gel. Plasmid DNA clones containing
176 and ~150 bp DNA insert respectively were grown to large scale and
purified on a Quigen column before sequencing. Both the strands were
sequenced using forward and reverse sequencing primer from the kit
(Sequenase Version 2, Amersham). Sequences of the plasmid having an insert
of ~150 bp is shown which reads the sequence form 5' to 3' direction of the
coding strand. Exact location and extent of the deletion is also shown. Plasmid
with 176 bp DNA fragment showed wild-type CCR5 sequences (Samson et
al., Z1996b) (data not shown).

could be easily identified. As expected 176 bp DNA fragment was identified
in all the individuals but only one individual showed about 150 bp additional
DNA band (Fig. 1, lane 2). Lanes 1, 3 and 4 show the PCR profile of three
other normal unrelated individuals and lane 5 shows the PCR amplified DNA
when pCCR5 plasmid DNA (Kind gift from Marc parmentier, Belgium).
Lane M represents the PCR marker lane with their sizes indicated on the right
side of the figure. This gel is a representative gel showing PCR analysis of
few individuals.

Cloning and Sequencing of PCR Amplified CCR5 Fragments

We cloned the 176 (wild-type) and 144 bp fragment (Fig. 1, lane 2) into a T-tailed vector (pGEM-T-Easy) and purified the plasmid DNAs on a Qiagen column before subjecting them to sequencing. A precise 32 bp. deletion corresponding to the second extracellular loop of the chemokine receptor was confirmed by sequencing (Fig. 2). Plasmid harboring the 176 bp CCR5 DNA fragment exhibited wild-type sequences only (data not shown).

Cloning of the Full Length CCR5 Gene (Wild type and Mutant) from the same Heterozygous Individual

A new set of primers were synthesized, one of which (5′ sense) overlapped the ATG initiation codon keeping the sequence in the strong Kozak context and the other primer was from the 3′ untranslated region of the gene (antisense primer). They had the following sequence:

(1) 5′- aagatggattatcaagtgtcaag
(2) 5′- ctcgtcgacatgtgccacaactctgactg

This primer combination (referred to as second set) is expected to amplify a 1 Kb CCR5 fragment. The amplified fragments from the heterozygous individual was cloned into pGEM-T-Easy and individual clones checked for the insert by *EcoR*1 and *Bgl* II digestion. The wild type clone could be easily identified from the mutant clone by 4% agarose gel analysis where a 32 base pair deleted fragment could be easily identified (Fig. 3, compare lane 1 with lane 2). Lanes 3 and 4 are molecular weight marker lanes (see legends to the figure). The corecptor functions were studied as described by us earlier (Husain et al., 1998) using recombinant vaccinia virus (Fuerst et al., 1987 and Banerjea et al., 1988 and Banerjea and Joklik, 1990). It was found out that the mutant CCR5 had a moderate effect on the wild-type coreceptor activity by cell fusion assay (data not shown).

Improved Genotyping by PCR and Restriction Enzymes

A 1 Kb fragment was amplified by PCR directly from the genomic DNAs of normal healthy individuals including the heterozygous (for Δ32 deletion mutant allele of CCR5) using the second set of primers and subjecting 1/10th of this material directly to *EcoR1* and Bgl II digestion using medium salt buffer conditions. The digestion products were then analyzed on a 4% agarose gel. Heterozygous individuals could be easily identified from a wild-type individual by exhibiting an additional DNA band (4 DNA bands in the heterozygous individual as compared to 3 common DNA bands in the wild-type individual) (Fig. 4).

Conclusions on the CCR5 Genotyping of Normal Healthy Indians

Our study brings out a very significant finding that the incidence of this

Genotyping of CCR5 gene by PCR & Restriction enzymes

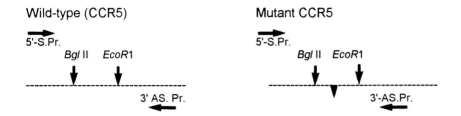

Wild-type (CCR5)   Mutant CCR5

PCR amplified 1099 bp DNA Clone into
pGem-T- Easy and subject individual clones to

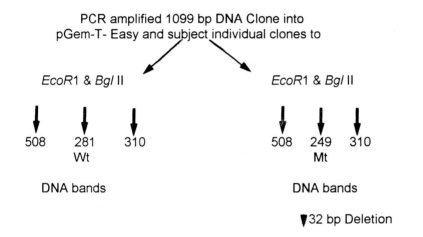

EcoR1 & Bgl II   EcoR1 & Bgl II

508   281   310   508   249   310
       Wt   Mt

DNA bands   DNA bands

▼32 bp Deletion

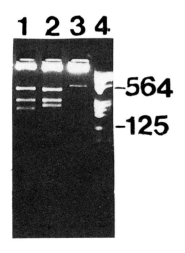

1 2 3 4

−564

−125

Fig. 3. A and B. The CCR5 gene analysis by restriction enzymes. Approximately 1 Kb CCR5 fragment was amplified by PCR using the genomic DNA of sample # 5 (Fig. 1, lane 2), and cloned into pGEM-T-Easy as described before. The clones were first confirmed to possess 1 Kb DNA insert and then subjected it to *EcoR*1 and *Bg/*II digestion. Mt CCR5 gene could be easily identified by analyzing the restriction fragments on a 4% agarose gel (3A). A faster migrating band of 249 bp (lane 1) could easily be identified from a wild type DNA band of 281 bp (lane 2). Lane 3 (λ/HindIII marker) and 4 (OX174/ HaeIII) show molecular weights of DNA standards. Note that in a 4% gel, any DNA above 1 Kb does not enter and stays at the top of the loading well (3B).

Genotyping of CCR5 gene by PCR & Restriction enzymes

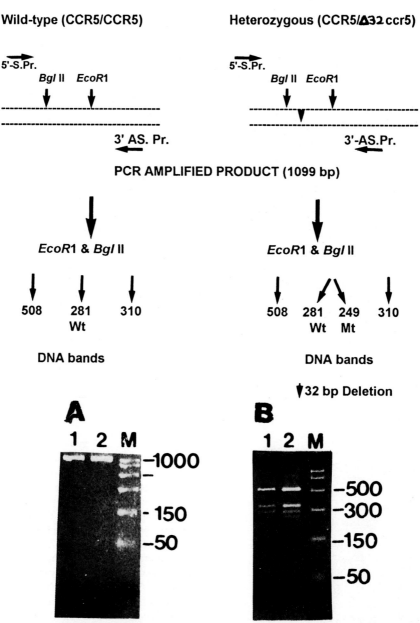

Fig. 4. Genotyping of CCR5 gene by PCR and restriction enzymes. After isolating genomic DNA from peripheral blood lymphocytes, the primer pair designed to amplify about 1 Kb (corresponds to the entire coding region) of CCR5 fragment (panel A, lanes 1 and 2. Thereafter, a small fraction (1/10th volume) of this PCR product is directly subjected to restriction enzyme digestion with E*co*R1 and *Bgl* II. A heterozygous individual could be easily identified from a person with wild type allele for CCR5 by observing an additional DNA band of 249 base pair (compare lanes 1 and 2 of panel B) when analyzed on a 4% agarose gel.

mutant allele (Δ32) is likely to be very low in India. This is in sharp contrast to the situation in Caucasian population of European heritage where heterozygous (for the Δ32 allele) is to the extent of 15 to 20% among normal unrelated individuals. A complete absence of a homozygous deletion among normal healthy Indians could have very significant implications in HIV-1 spread and infection. It is noteworthy that about 1% Caucasian population is homozygous for this deletion allele. This may partially explain as to why in India and in Asia the HIV-1 is spreading at an alarming rate.

Ribozymes

Construction of Ribozymes against Chemokine Receptore-CCR5 gene

Since individuals with homozygous deletion in the CCR5 gene are healthy and physically fit, this gene has become target for intervention. We have constructed a monoribozyme with a hammer-head motif that cleaves the CCR5 gene specifically in a Mg^{++} dependent and protein independent manner. We wish to selectively down regulate the expression of CCR5 RNA in side the cell with the hope that the macrophage-tropic isolates of HIV-1 will not be able to infect the cell. Figure 5 shows precise cleavage of the CCR5 RNA by ribozymes in presence of two different concentrations of $MgCl_2$ (2 and 10 mM) and two kinds of temerature conditions for cleavage. In one case the substrate and ribozyme were allowed to interact with ribozyme entirely at 37°C (Fig. 5, lanes 2 and 3) and in the other case, heating at 90°C preceded the incubation at 37°C (lane 4 and 5). Note the cleavage only in presence of

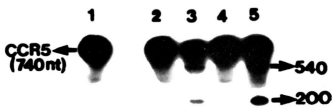

Fig. 5. *In vitro* **cleavage of CCR5 gene by ribozyme. Labeled** *in vitro* **transcript were generated by T7 RNA polymerase by first digesting the CCR5 gene by *Bgl* IIenzyme (expected to generate 740 bp RNA) and cold ribozyme targeted to cleave at 541 nucleotide of CCR5 gene. Equimolar concentration of ribozyme and substrate RNA were mixed and cleavage reaction was initiated by adding 2-10 mM $MgCl_2$. Lane 1 shows the formation of 740 bases long RNA. Lanes 2 and 3 show the cleavage carried out at 37°C at 2 and 10 mM $MgCl_2$ concentration respectively. Note the precise cleavage products in lane 3. Lane 4 and 5 show the cleavage carried out by first heating the substrate and ribozyme at 90°C for 3 min followed by 2 hours at 37°C in presence of 2 mM and 10 mM $MgCl_2$ concentration respectively. Note the precise cleavage of CCR5 RNA in lane 5. Two conclusions can be drawn. Cleavage at 10 mM $MgCl_2$ was significantly better than 2 mM and additional heating improves the cleavage efficiency only marginally.**

10 mM $MgCl_2$ (lanes 3 and 5). Lane 1 shows the synthesis of 740 bases long CCR5 transcript.

DNA-Enzyme Against HIV-1 Env Gene

DNA-enzyme against HIV-1 Env has been assembled by standard procedures (Chen-Banerjea et al., 1992 and Paik-Banerjea et al., 1997) using the recently identified 10–23 catalytic motif. The cleavage site was present at the 6339 nucleotide position (AUG) of the infectious clone of HIV-1 (pNL4–3, Adachi et al., 1986). Precise cleavage of the target RNAs were again observed in a Mg^{++} dependent manner. Figure 6 shows the cleavage of the HIV envelope gene by DNA-enzyme only in presence of Mg++ (lanes 4 and 5) into specific 5′ and 3′ cleaved products. No cleavage was observed in absence of Mg++ (lane 2), very little cleavage was obtained at 0.1 mM $MgCl_2$ (lane 2). HIV-1 specific trucated Envelope (180 nt) was synthesized under *in vitro* conditions (lane 1).

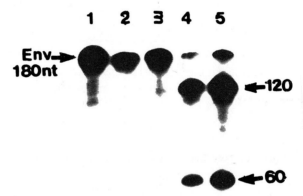

Fig. 6.   Cleavage by DNA-enzyme. Lane 1 shows the 180 bp labeled transcript of HIV-1 Env (III B strain) that was synthesized *in vitro* by T7 RNA polymearse (Promega Biotech., USA). DNA-enzyme with 10–23 catalytic motif failed to cleave the transcript in absence of Mg^{++} (lane 2), very inefficient cleavage in presence of 1mM $MgCl_2$ (lane 3) but more than 80–90% specific cleavage was obtained in presence of 10 mM (lane 4) and 20 mM $MgCl_2$ concentration. It can be concluded that DNA-enzyme is functional in its ability to cleave HIV-1 env RNA in a sequence specific manner.

Conclusions on Ribozymes and DNA-enzyme

Ribozymes that have the ability to cleave precisely the various HIV-1 genes and the HIV-1 coreceptor gene (CCR5) have been constructed by recombinant means. Efforts are being made to selectively down regulate these genes intracellularly with the purpose of down regulating the replication of HIV-1 in a susceptible host cell. Precise cleavage of the HIV-1 envelope gene was obtained by mono-DNA-enzyme.

References

Adachi, A., Glendelman, H.E., Koenig, S., Folks, T., Willey, R., Rabsom, A., and Martin, M. 1986. Production of acquired immunodeficiency syndrome associated retrovirus in human and nonhuman cells transfected with an infectious molecular clone. *J. Virol.* **59:** 284–291.

Banerjea, A.C., Kedarnath, N., Gore, M.M. Dayaraj, C.C., Jamkar, A.V., and Ghosh, S.N. 1981. Interferon (type α and γ) production by fresh and cryopreserved human mononuclear cells. *Arch. Virol.* **69:** 91–914.

Banerjea, A.C., Brechling, K., Ray, C.A., Erickson, H., Pickup, D.J., Joklik, W.K. 1988. High-level synthesis of biologically active reovirus protein $\sigma1$ in a mammalian expression vector system. *Virology* **167:** 601–612.

Banerjea, A.C., and Joklik, W.K. 1990. Reovirus protein $\sigma1$ translated in vitro, as well as truncated derivatives of it that lack up to two-thirds of its C-terminal portion, exists as two major tetramolecular species that differ in electrophoretic mobility. *Virology* **179:** 460–462.

Bitti et al. 1997. HIV-1 infection in an individual homozygous for the CCR5 deletion allele. *Nature Medicine* **3:** 252–253.

Chen, C-J., Banerjea, A.C., Harmison, G.G., Haglund, K., Schubert, M. 1992. Multitarget-ribozyme directed to cleave up to nine highly conserved HIV-1 env RNA regions inhibits HIV-1 replication—potential effectiveness against most presently sequenced HIV-1 isolates. *Nucleic Acids Research* **20:** 4581–4589.

D'Souza, M.P., Harde, A.V. 1996. Chemokines and HIV-1 second receptors. *Nature Medicine* **2:** 1293–1300.

Fuerst, T.R., Earl, P.L., Moss, B. 1987. Use of hybrid vaccinia virus-T7 polymerase system for expression of target genes. *Mol. Cell. Biol.* **7:** 2538–2544.

He., et al., 1997. CCR3 and CCR5 are coreceptors for HIV-1 infection of microglia. *Nature* **385:** 645–649.

Huang et al. 1996. The role of mutant CCR5 allele in HIV-1 transmission and disease progression. *Nature Medicine* **2:** 1240–1243.

Husain, S., Goila, R., Shahi, S., Banerjea, A.C. 1998. First report of a healthy Indian heterozygous for Δ32 mutant of HIV-1 coreceptor-CCR5. *Gene* **207:** 141–147.

Liu et al. 1996. Homozygous defect in HIV-1 coreceptor accounts for resistance of some multiply exposed individuals to HIV-1 infection. *Cell* **86:** 367–377.

Paik, S-Y., Banerjea, A., Chen, C.-J., Ye, Z., harmison, G.G., Schubert, M. 1997. Defective HIV-1 provirus encoding a multi-target ribozyme inhibits accumulation of spliced and unspliced HIV-1 mRNAs, reduces infectivity of viral progeny, and protects the cells from pathogenesis. *Human Gene Therapy* **8:** 1115–1124.

Paik, S-Y., Banerjea, A.C., Harmison, G.G., Chen, C.-J., Schubert, M. 1995. Inducible and conditional inhibition of human immunodeficiency virus proviral expression by vesicular stomatitis virus matrix protein. *J. Virol.* **69:** 3529–3537.

Immunopharmacology: Strategies for immunotherapy
S.N. Upadhyay (Ed)

3. DNA Binding Protein HLP_{Mt} of *Mycobacterium tuberculosis:* A target of human immune response

**P. Savita[1], K. Raha[1], P.S. Annapurna[1], S. Kaur[1], N. Islam[1],
S. Zzaman[1], M. Raje[2], A.B. Dey[3], N.K. Jain[4], V. Kothekar[5],
J.S. Tyagi[1] and H.K. Prasad[1]**

[1]Dept. of Biotechnology, All India Institute of Medical Sciences,
New Delhi-110029, India

[2]Institute of Microbial Technology, Chandigarh-160014, India

[3]Dept. of Medicine, All India Institute of Medical Sciences, New Delhi-110029, India

[4]New Delhi Tuberculosis Centre, New Delhi-110002, India

[5]Dept. of Biophysics, All India Institute of Medical Sciences, New Delhi-110029, India

Abstract

An immuno-subtractive procedure was adopted to identify a 30-kDa antigen of mycobacteria associated with human immune response. Transblots of sonicated *M. tuberculosis* (MTB) were incubated with murine monoclonal antibodies specific for mycobacterial antigens, followed by human sera derived from healthy contacts and patients. All sera showed persistent reactivity with proteins of MTB in the molecular weight range of 30 kDa and less. The predominant 30-kDa protein was purified and used for generation of murine monospecific sera. The protein is not secreted into the extracellular culture fluid as seen in immunoblots and ELISA assays, hence differs from all other secretory proteins of mycobacteria hitherto described in a similar molecular weight range. Using immuno-gold electron microscopy our results demonstrate for the first time the direct evidence of the restricted distribution of a 30-kDa mycobacterial protein in the cytosolic compartment of mycobacteria. The protein is immunogenic and is capable of inducing *in vitro* lymphoproliferation in tuberculin reactors.

A 3-dimensional model of this protein was built based on its primary structure, using homology based modelling tools available on the Internet. This was followed by energy optimisation using molecular mechanics and dynamics technique on INDIGO II-R-4400 extreme graphics workstation. The protein in association with 35 base paired GC rich U bend-DNA complex was simulated using Amber 4.0 molecular dynamics package. The protein appears to be involved in packaging and stabilisation of DNA.

Introduction

M. tuberculosis induces humoral as well as cell mediated immune response in infected humans and experimental animals. Several antigenic immune components have been characterised using murine monoclonal antibodies [1]. It has been the goal of several laboratories to characterise the complex mycobacterial constituents, with an aim to identify unique antigens associated with human immune response. We have identified a mycobacterial protein by using the strategy of subtractive immunoblotting. This protein is not secreted into the extracellular medium and therefore, is different from the hitherto described mycobacterial antigens in a 30-kDa molecular weight range such as antigens of the 85 ABC complex [2, 3]. This is the first report of a mycobacterial antigen, which is exclusively confined to the cytosolic compartment of the tubercle bacilli.

Materials and Methods

Subjects: Serum samples were collected from two groups of individuals: (i) Healthy residents of endemic areas/who had close contact with patients, (ii) 25 patients of pulmonary tuberculosis attending New Delhi Tuberculosis Centre. Prior to inclusion in the study, the contacts were screened for clinical signs and symptoms of tuberculosis. Twentysix of them were tuberculin reactive.

Antigens: *M. tuberculosis* (H37 Rv and H37 Ra) (Tuberculosis Research Centre, Madras, India) and *M. bovis* BCG (Japan BCG lab, Tokyo) cultured in. *Kirchner's* medium [4] were heat killed and harvested. The washed mycobacterial pellet was suspended in TBS (50 mM, 150 mM NaCl, pH 7.2) containing 1 mM phenylmethylsulfonyl fluoride sigma, St. Louis, USA), dithiothreitol (Sigma, St. Louis, USA), EDTA (Sigma, St. Louis, USA) and 10 mM 2-mercaptoethanol (Sigma, St. Louis, USA). The bacterial suspension was sonicated. The protein concentration of the sonic extract was determined by standard techniques [5]. The corresponding MTB culture supernates were filtered (0.45 μm, Millipore, USA) and concentrated and used as a source of secreted antigens.

Monoclonal and Polyclonal Antibodies: Monoclonal antibodies specific for antigens of *M. tuberculosis* were kindly provided by The IMMTUB bank of The World Health Organisation and by Drs D. Chatterjee (Colorado state University, Fort Collins, Colorado, USA), D.B. Young (St. Mary's Hospital Medical School, London, UK). Transblots of mycobacterial proteins separated by SDS-PAGE were probed with these antibodies, using standard immunoblotting techniques. Prof. M. Harboe, (Institute of Rheumatology,

Oslo, Norway.) kindly provided the rabbit sera specific for the 85A, B and C antigens of mycobacteria.

SDS-PAGE, Immunoblotting: The resolved mycobacterial proteins (Fig. 1A) were electroblotted on to nitro-cellulose (Millipore, USA) (6). The nonspecific binding sites were blocked by incubation with 1% reconstituted dried skimmed milk powder (Anik Spray, Gujarat, India) in TBS (0.1 m, pH 7.2). Membranes were cut into vertical strips. The strips were incubated with individual plasma/sera (1:100), at room temperature. After washing the strips were incubated with peroxidase conjugated rabbit anti-human IgG (gamma chain, Dakopatts, Denmark 1:500) for 30 mins. The strips were washed and exposed to substrate solution, (6 mg 4-chloro-napthol, (Sigma), The reaction was terminated after appropriate intensity of colour development.

Detection of Mycobacterial Antigens Unique to Human Immune Response: Blocked transblots were treated as follows: each strip was treated initially

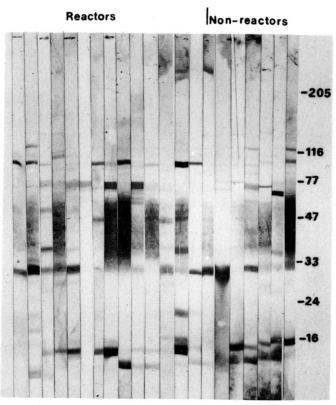

Fig. 1A. Representative immunoblots of *M. tuberculosis* sonic extract probed with sera/plasma (1:100 dilution) of healthy non-tuberculous contacts. Position of molecular weight markers is indicated on the right. Tuberculin reactors (Lanes 1-13); tuberculin non-reactors (Lanes 14–20).

with murine monoclonal antibodies specific for MTB antigens at the recommended dilutions followed by exposure to human sera (1:100). The binding of human antibodies was visualised using peroxidase conjugated to anti-human lgG and the appropriate substrate.

Relationship of 30 kDa Antigens with 85 ABC Complex: Electroblots of *M. bovis* (BCG) sonicates were blocked as before and the corresponding culture filtrate were probed with rabbit antisera specific for the antigens of the 85 ABC complex (1 : 200, kind gift of Prof. Morten Harboe) and anti-30 kDa antibodies generated as ascitic fluid in mice (1:200).

Electron Microscopic Localisation of 30-kDa Antigen by Immunogold Labelling: Immunolabeling of ultrathin sections of *M. tuberculosis* was done as described by Varndeell and Polak [7]. Actively growing cultures of MTB were harvested. The mycobacterial pellet was fixed, serially dehydrated and embedded in Pure LR white resin (London Resin Co., England). After Polymerisation, ultrathin sections were cut. The sections were mounted on to nickel grids (Bio-rad). The mounted grids were processed for immunogold labelling as follows; the grids were treated with membrane filtered (0.22 μm) blocking solution (3% BSA in PBS, 20 mM pH 7.4) for 30 mins. The washed grids were incubated with 1:10 dilution of the murine 30 kDa antibody followed by the second antibody (Rabbit anti-mouse 250 ng/ml). The grids were finally treated with Protein A gold (1:100, particle size 10 nm, Sigma). The washed grids were stained with 3% aqueous uranyl acetate (Sigma) and viewed using a Jeol model Transmission Electron microscope (Japan). Control grids were treated with ascitic fluid derived from unimmunized mice.

Antigens for the Lymphoproliferative Assay: The following antigens were used in the study: (a) Nitro-cellulose (NC) strips devoid of antigen (Negative control), (b) Twenty microgram protein of the sonic MTB extract was adsorbed on to a nitro-cellulose strip (4 × 120 mm) (positive control, MTB-NC); (c) The 30 kDa antigen of *M. tuberculosis* (30 kDa-NC). The 30-kDa antigen was identified using the murine monospecific sera as described earlier. The relevant nitro-cellulose strip was cut and the bound antigens of MTB were processed as described by Abou-Zeid [6]. The nitro-cellulose bound antigens and nitro-cellulose devoid of antigen (Negative Control) were dissolved in minimal quantities of dimethyl-sulfoxide (Sigma) and re-precipitated with equal volume of carbonate-bicarbonate buffer (50 mM, pH 9.6). The particles were washed thrice with RPM 1-1640 (GIBCO, Scotland, UK) containing 25 mM HEPES, 100 units of penicillin/ml (Alembic Chemical Works, Vadodara, India), 100 μg of streptomycin/ml (Synbiotics Ltd., Vadodara, India), by centrifuging at 5000 g for 30 mins. The pellets were resuspended in 1ml RPM1-1640, aliquoted and stored at −70°C. For the proliferative assay 25 μl of the suspension (1:50) was added to a microtiter containing 10^5 peripheral blood mononuclear cells (PBMC).

Lymphoproliferative Assay: PBMC were isolated from peripheral blood by ficoll gradient [8]. The cells were suspended in 10% human AB serum-RPMI-1640 media. One hundred microliters of the fluid containing 10^5 of cells was distributed into 96 well plates (Linbro, UK). For each donor the proliferative assay was set up in quadruplicates, as follows: (i) PBMC alone, (ii) +25 μl of NC, (iii) +MTB-NC, (iv) +30 kDa-NC. The plates were incubated at 37°C, in a 5% CO_2 atmosphere for five days and ^{3}H-thymidine specific activity 1Ci/mmol was added to each well (BRIT, Bombay, India) on the fifth day. After an additional sixteen hours incubation, the cells were harvested on to glass fibre filter paper strips (Whatman, USA) with a cell harvester (PHD Cell Harvester, Cambridge Inc., MA, USA), dried and processed for liquid scintillation counting (LKB Rack beta counter, Turku, Finland, 40% efficiency for ^{3}H isotope). The antigen-driven proliferative results have been expressed as stimulation index (S.I.) with the background responses to nitro-cellulose alone (NC, control) deducted, stimulation indices being the ratio of the counts per minute (cpm) in the stimulated cultures vs cpm in control cultures. Stimulation index of 2 or more was considered as positive response.

Computer Modelling Techniques: Secondary structure prediction of the protein was carried out using programs: predict, PHD, Chou & Fasman, C, F & Rose, Gibrat, Levin, DPM, SOPM, PSSP on predict-protein server http://www.Embl-heidelberg./predict. Consensus from these studies was used for secondary structure assignment of HLP_{Mt}. Definitive regions of prediction by PHD were given maximum weightage. Multiple sequence alignment was done using Max Hom, Predict.Protein server. The BLASTP search yielded score of 218 for 1HUE (*Bacillus stearothermophilus*) following this both chains of IHF (Integration Host Factor of *E. coli*) having a score of 169 and 122, respectively, for the first ninety residues. The residues after this showed mainly helical confirmation and did not have homology with any known protein structure. Hence homology based modelling was done using Swiss Model on Expasy Server using structures of 1HUE (9–11) and IHF (12). The secondary structure assignment of HLP_{Mt} is shown in Table 1. The structure of the protein was energy minimised by AMBER 4.0 (13) on INDIGO-II, R-4400 extreme graphics work station.

The structure of IHF was available with a 35 base paired U-bend nicked DNA. Since there was no other report on structure of complex of histone like protein with DNA, we took this structure as a starting model. IHF DNA had a nick at the 14th base pair. We first corrected its nick using in house package MODEL. Next, as the *M. tuberculosis* genome is rich in GC base pairs, the nucleotides in close contact with protein were replaced by GC base pairs. Structure of the complex HLP_{Mt} with U-bend DNA (U_{35} DNA) was obtained by in house docking program IMF1. The complex was energy minimised by AMBER 4.0 [13]. Molecular dynamics simulation of HLP_{Mt} (first ninety-one residues), U_{35} DNA and complex of HLP_{Mt} with U_{35} DNA was done using

MINMD module of AMBER 4.0 using united atom force field (where hydrogen atoms attached to carbon are neglected) of Cornell *et al.* [14], distance dependent di-electric constant, time step of 0.001 pico seconds (ps), with cut-off distance for non-bonded pair list of 8 Å and the pair list upgraded after 20 cycles. The simulation was carried out for 250 ps after equilibration at 310°. The MD trajectories were analysed using MOLMOL of Koradi [15], PCURVES by Lavery & Sklenar, [16, 17] and in house package ANALMD. Several geometry dependent parameters were calculated.

Table 1. Secondary structural elements in HLP_{Mt}. For comparison we have also shown the same of 1 HUE as obtained by x-ray crystallography [9] and NMR spectroscopy [11].

Secondary structure	Residue HLP_{mt}	Residue HU-crys [9]	Residue HU-nmr [11]
$\alpha 1$	4–14	3–13	4–14
$\alpha 2$	18–36	21–37	18–39
$\alpha 3$	83–89	84–89	84–89
$\beta 1$	42–44	40–44	41–45
$\beta 2$	48–55	48–51	48–52
$\beta 3$	58–62	—	53–56
$\beta 4$	67–71	—	73–76
$\beta 5$	74–81	78–83	77–81
Turn 1	15–17		
Turn 2	37–41		
Turn 3	45–47		
Turn 4	63–65		

Results

Identification of Antigens of *M. tuberculosis* Associated with Human Immune Response

A two-step strategy was employed to identify antigens of *M. tuberculosis* uniquely reactive with human antibodies. Initially transblots of *M. tuberculosis* were exposed to a panel of characterised murine monoclonal antibodies against mycobacterial antigens (IMMTUB, WHO). In the second step, these blots were exposed to individual sera/pools of sera derived from healthy contacts (15 reactors and 10 non-reactors) and 10 patients. Comparing the immuno-reactivity of the sera in Fig. 1A with the reactivity seen in Fig. 1B and B′ it appears that the human and murine antibody response was similar to mycobacterial antigens in the molecular weight range of 71-35 kDa. However reactivity was also seen for antigens of 16, 17–19 and 30 kDa, indicating that these antigens were unique to human antibody response. Regardless of the source of the sera/pool of sera, predominant persistent immuno-reactivity was seen with mycobacterial antigens in the mol. wt of 30 kDa and less (Fig. 1, B and B′). This antigen was taken up for further study.

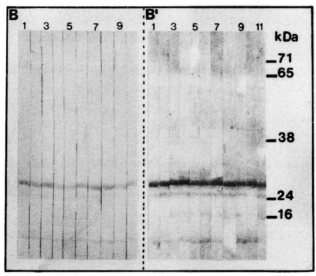

Fig. 1.   B, B′. Subtractive Immunoblot: Representative immunoblot probed for the binding of human sera on transblots initially treated with murine monoclonal antibodies. Note the persistent immunoreactivity with human sera in the 30 kDa region and less. The molecular weight markers are indicated on the right. 1B: Lanes 1-10 exposed to non-tuberculous healthy contacts (1-5 tuberculin reactors, 6-10 non-reactors).

Relationship of 30 kDa Antigens with 85 ABC Complex

Immuno-reactivity of the monospecific sera was limited to sonic extracts of *M. bovis*. No reactivity was detected with the corresponding culture filtrate antigen (Fig. 2A). Simultaneously blots were probed with rabbit sera specific for the secretory antigens of the 85 ABC complex of mycobacteria. The 3 components have molecular weights in the range of 30-32 kDa [2]. The antigens were detected both in the culture filtrate and sonic extracts. Therefore the 30 kDa antigen is distinct from the secreted 85 complex of antigens (Fig. 2A).

Localisation of 30 kDa Antigen: ELISA assays with sonicates and integral bacilli of *M. tuberculosis* and monospecific sera for the 30 kDa antigen was carried out. The reactivity was seen exclusively with sonic extracts of tubercle bacilli and was not detected with integral bacilli (Fig. 3).

Intracellular Localisation of the 30 kDa antigen

In order to establish the sub-cellular distribution of the 30-kDa antigen, immunogold labelling was carried out. Ultrathin sections of the tubercle bacilli were treated serially with anti-30 kDa antibody, anti-mouse rabbit sera and protein gold (10 nm gold particle size). While staining the control grids, the 1st antibody was replaced with ascitic fluid derived from unimmunized mice.

On scanning the probed grids the gold particles were seen only in bacillary sections treated immune sera (Fig. 4, B and C). Rarely One/two particles were seen non-specifically located in the embedding resin in the control sections or at sites of discontinuity in the cell wall (Fig. 4A). The gold particles were distributed randomly in the cytosol (Fig. 4B) as well along the cytoplasmic face of the wall of the bacillus (Fig. 4C). The gold labelling was absent on the surface of the mycobacterial cell. The distribution of the gold particles on randomly photographed bacilli was enumerated. Ninetyone percent of the gold particles were found to be associated with the bacilli (Fig. 4B). Occasionally 4–6 gold particles/bacilli were seen (Fig. 3, B and C). In some bacilli the gold particles were present in clusters.

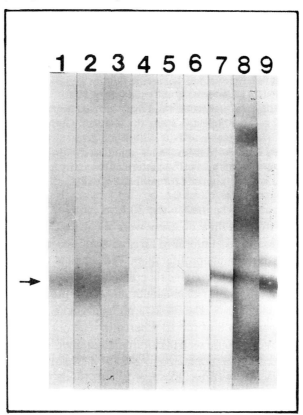

Fig. 2. Comparative analysis of the distribution of the 30 kDa antigen with antigens of the 85 ABC complex in *M. bovis* (BCG). Immunoblot of sonic extract (lanes 6–9) and culture filtrate (lane 1–4) of BCG probed with monospecific sera for 30 kDa (lanes 4, 6) and 85 A, B and C antigens (lanes 1–3, 7–9). Antigen 85A (lanes 1, 7), B (lanes 2, 8) and C (lanes 3, 9) were detected both in sonic extract and culture filtrate. The 30 kDa antigen was detected only in sonicate (lane 6).

The results of the immuno-electron microscopy provide the direct evidence of the intracellular location of the 30 kDa antigen in tubercle bacilli, confirming

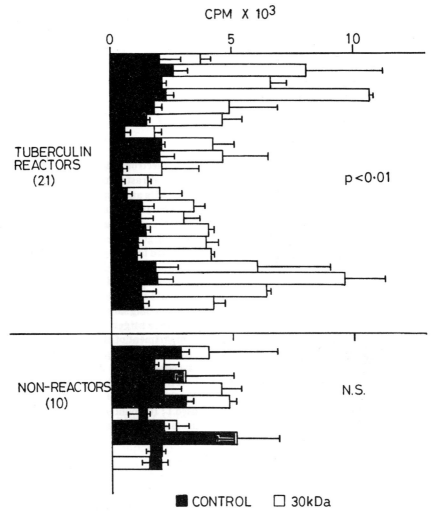

Fig. 5. Histogram depicting the proliferative responses of PBMC derived from healthy non-tuberculous individuals after *in vitro* stimulation with the 30 kDa mycobacterial antigen bound to nitro-cellulose. The extent of proliferation was assessed by the incorporation of [³H] thymidine into the cultured mononuclear cells. The mean radioactive counts of quadruplicate culture for each individual have been represented as histograms and S.D. as bars (mean cpm ±S.D.). Upper panel shows the response of 21 tuberculin reactors; lower panel 10 non-reactors. (Control cultures devoid of antigen; 30 kDa antigen stimulated cultures) (p value of 30 kDa cultures vs controls < 0.01; N.S.: not significant).

of the U_{35} DNA. The arm region and the $\alpha 3$ of HLP_{Mt} interact with the bridge of the DNA. The core region helices ($\alpha 1$ and $\alpha 2$) are hydrophobic in nature interact with the arms of the U_{35} DNA. These results suggest, that the mycobacterial protein HLP_{Mt} may be involved in compaction, packaging and stabilisation of DNA structure.

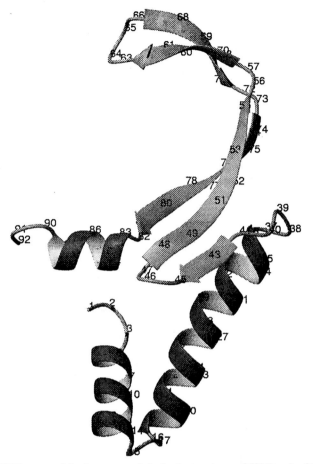

Fig. 6. Ribbon model of energy minimised structure of HLP$_{Mt}$ by MOLMOL.

Discussion

Using murine monoclonal antibodies several mycobacterial proteins have been isolated and have been shown to be recognised by the human immune system [1]. However, this does not encompass the spectrum of antigens recognised by humans or the antigenic challenge encountered by infected individuals [1, 19, 26]. The reasons for this could stem from the fact that humans are naturally infected with live organisms unlike mice deliberately immunised with heat killed/indicated mycobacteria. These antigenic preparations do not represent the gamut of antigens generated by live mycobacteria *in vivo*. Experiments related to the induction of resistance in mice lend credence to the fact that live bacilli as opposed to killed mycobacteria induce protection [24]. Further, the perception of mycobacterial antigens by the human immune system may differ from the murine system. Isolation and characterisation of these unique antigens would be useful for designing of diagnostic/therapeutic reagents.

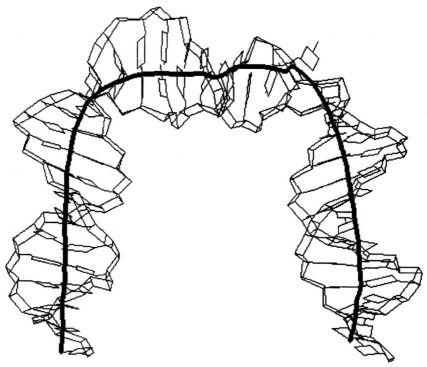

Fig. 7.   Backbone of U_{35} DNA using P-CURVES [16, 17].

In this paper we report the characterisation of a mycobacterial antigen associated with human immune response and its localisation *in situ* in tubercle bacilli.

The precise topographical distribution and location of immunogenic constituents would help in the understanding of their involvement in host-mycobacterial interaction or their physiological role in mycobacteria. Immuno-gold electron microscopic technique has been extensively used to establish the exact location of several immuno-reactive antigens of mycobacteria. For example, Lamb has been localised on the mycobacterial cell surface as a loose capsular material [20, 27]. Some components have been shown to be distributed on the cell surface and cell wall as in the case of the fibronectin binding protein 29–33 kDa, [21] and the phosphate binding protein 38-kDa [25]. Or in the cytoplasm as has been reported in case of the 65-kDa heat shock protein [22].

Our study is the first report to demonstrate the direct evidence of localisation of a mycobacterial protein in the molecular weight range of 30 kDa that is confined in its distribution within the cytosolic compartment of the mycobacterial cell. In the cytoplasm the gold particles were seen randomly distributed either as discrete particles or in clusters. Occasionally the gold particles were seen localised along the cytoplasmic surface of the mycobacterial cell wall. Studies are underway to localise this antigen during various growth

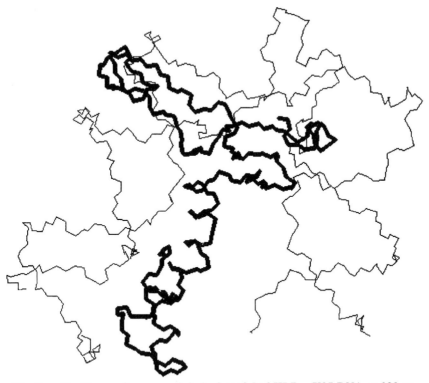

Fig. 8a.   Backbone of energy minimised model of HLP$_{Mt}$ U35-DNA at 232 ps.

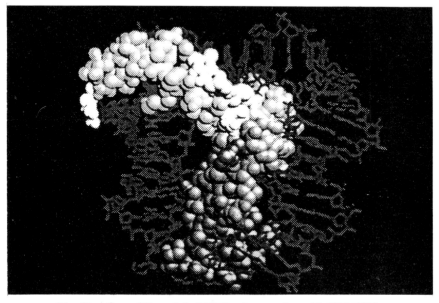

Fig. 8b.   Spacefill model of HLP$_{Mt}$ in complex with U35 DNA.

phases of mycobacteria. The 30-kDa protein described in this study is not secreted unlike proteins in a similar molecular weight range such as the 85 ABC antigen complex. Thus there exists a characteristic difference in the distribution and location of the 30-kDa antigen compared with other mycobacterial antigens reported in literature.

We also provide preliminary evidence of the involvement of this protein in cell medicated immune response in healthy non-tuberculous contacts (Fig. 5). The 30 kDa protein induces significant proliferation in tuberculin reactors, while no induction of lymphoproliferation was observed in non-reactors to tuberculin.

The presence of this protein exclusively in the cytoplasm combined with its non-secretory nature make it a useful marker to monitor mycobacterial lysis mediated *in vitro* by immunological mechanisms or by anti-mycobacterial drugs. Proteins such as Gorel/65 kDa and iso-citrate dehydrogenase have been shown to be released during autolysis [2, 22, 23]. However these proteins are homologous to host cell derived proteins such as the 65 kDa protein a member of the stress related proteins and iso-citrate dehydrogenase, an enzyme of the TCA cycle. Therefore these proteins cannot be used as markers of mycobacterial lysis *in vivo* or *in vitro*. The 30 kDa cytoplasmic protein antigen or mycobacteria described in this study is an ideal candidate to be used as a marker to detect lysis of pathogenic mycobacteria. The protein when released from its natural environment is stable as indicated by the presence of circulating antibodies and antigen reactive lymphocytes in healthy individuals. However its potential utility *in vivo* studies will need to be critically evaluated.

As no structural data was available for HLP_{Mt} we followed a systemic approach of predicting the structure from amino acid sequence, homology based modelling, and using co-ordinates of homologous proteins (1HUE, IHF) from the Protein Data Bank (PDB), to obtain the three dimensional structure of the first 90 residues of HLP_{Mt}. A model for its complex with 35 base paired, GC rich, U-bent DNA (U_{35} DNA) was obtained using the only available structure of histone like proteins (IHF) with DNA. The GC rich DNA model was created in keeping with the GC rich nature of genome of *M. tuberculosis* and the conformation usually seen with DNA binding proteins. The (U_{35} DNA) HLP_{Mt} complex was optimised by molecular mechanics and molecular dynamics method using AMBER.4.0 package.

We found that, in the absence of the HLP_{Mt} protein the U35-DNA straightens out. However, in the presence of the protein, it undergoes compaction and super secondary structural changes. These changes were found to be dependent on the primary sequence of the protein and distribution of lysine and arginine residues. The protein also got stabilised in the presence of DNA. Therefore there appears to be an intricate functional and structural relationship between the DNA binding protein HLP_{Mt} and the DNA structure.

Further studies are being carried out to examine the interaction of the entire protein (214 amino acids) with GC rich mycobacterial DNA. Such studies will help in the designing of new therapeutic agents against novel mycobacterial targets. The study demonstrates the utility of adopting immunological techniques to identify, characterise unique mycobacterial antigens associated with human immune response.

Acknowledgements

The work has been supported by CSIR grant, DBT Govt. of India. Savita received the financial support from CSIR. Dr. Annapurana, Najmul, and Zzaman were Research Associates in the DBT Teaching program. The intellectual support of Drs. Indira Nath, A.K. Tyagi, S. Chauhan, S. Sinha and Bhavneet Singh Seerah for typing etc., and a host of others is acknowledged.

References

1. Young D.B., Kaufmann S.H.E., Hermans PWM, Thole JER. *Mol. Microbiol.* 1992; **6**: 133–145.
2. Wiker H.G., Harboe M. *Microbiol Rev.* 1992; **56**: 648–661.
3. Wiker H.G., Harboe M., Nagai S.A. *J. Gen Micribiol.* 1991; **173**: 875–884.
4. Mckee C.M., Rake G., Donovick R.P., Jambor W.P. *Am Rev Tuberc.* 1949; **60**: 90–108.
5. Bradford N.M. *Analytical Biochem.* 1976; **72**: 248–254.
6. Abou-Zeid C., Filley E., Steele J., Rook GAW. *J. Immunol Methods.* 1987; **98**: 5–10.
7. Varndell 1M., Polak J.M. Chapter 8. "EM Immunolabelling". In the entitled "Electron Microscopy in Molecular Biology, A practical Approach". Edited by Sommerville J, Sheer U. IRL press. 1987; 191–199.
8. Boyum A. Scand J. Clin Lab Invest. 1968; 21 (Suppl. 97) (paper-IV): 77–89.
9. Tanaka, L.K., Appelt, K., Disk J., White, S.W. and Wilson, K.S. *Nature.* 1984; **310**: 376–381.
10. White S.W., Appelt, K., Wilson K.S. and Tanaka, I. *Proteins.* 1959; **6**: 104–127.
11. Vis, H., Mariani, M. Vorgias, C.E., Wilson, K.S., Kaptein, K.S. and Boelens, R. *J. Mol. Biol.* 1995; 254, 692–703.
12. Rice, P.A., Yang, S.Y., Mizuuchi, K., and Nash, H.A. Cell 1996; 1295–1306.
13. Pearlman, D.A., Cald well, J.C., Singh U.C., Weiner, P.K. and Kollman P.A., Amber Y.O. 1993 A computer simulation software developed by University of California, USA.
14. Cornell, W.D., Cieplak, P., Bayly, C.L. Gold I.R., Merz, K.M., Feurgeueson, D.Y., Spellmeyer D.C., Fox, J. Caldwell, J.W., & Kollman, P.A. *J. Am. Chem. Soc.* 1995; **117**: 5179–519.
15. Koradi, R. 1997 MOLMOL—A molecular analysis and display program. Institute far Molecular Biology end Biophysics, EIH Zurich, Spectrospin, A.G., Fallenden Switzerland.
16. Lavery, R. and Sklenar, H. *J. Biomol. Struct. Dyn.* 1988; **6**: 63–91.
17. Lavery, R and Slelenor, H. *Structure and methods.* 1990; **2**: 215–235.
18. Sayle, R. 1994 RASMOL A molecular visualisation program of GLAXO Research and Development, Greenfield, Middle sex, UK.
19. Havlir D.V., Wallis S., Boom W.H., Thomas D.M., Chervenak K., Ellner J.J. *Infect Immun.* 1991; **59**: 665–670.

20. Hunter S.W., Brennan P.J., *J. Biol. Chem.* 1990; **265:** 9272–9279.
21. A Das P.K., Chand A., Baas J.G., Groothuis D.G., Kolk AHJ., Scad. *J. Immunol.* 1991; **33:** 765–775.
22. Rambukkana A., Das P.K., Burggraaf J.D., Faber W.R., Teeling P., Krieg S., Thole JER, Harboe M. *Infect Immun* 1992; **60:** 4517–4527.
23. Andersen P. Askgaard D., Ljungqvist L., Bentzon MW Heron. I. *Infect Immun.* 1991; **59:** 1558–1563.
24. Orme I. *Infect Immun.* 1988: **56:** 3310–312.
25. Espitila C., Elinos M., Pando R.H., Mancilla R. *Infect Immun.* 1992: **60:** 2998–3001.
26. Laal S., Samanich K.M., Sonnemberg M.G., Zolla-Pazner S., Phadtare J.M., and Belisle J.T. *Clin. Diagn. Lab. Immunol.* 1997; **4:** (In Press).
27. Boddingius J., and Dijkman H. *J. Gen. Micribiol.* 1990; **136:** 2001–2012.
28. Prabhakar S., Annapurna P.S., Jain N.K., Dey A.B., Tyagi J.S. and Prasad H.K. *Tub. and Lung Dis.* 1998 (In Press).

Immunopharmacology: Strategies for immunotherapy
S.N. Upadhyay (Ed)

4. NO: A versatile messenger involved in host defence

Jean-Claude Drapier

Institut de Chimie des Substances Naturelles, CNRS, 1, Avenue de la Terrasse,
91190 Gif-sur-Yvette, France

Summary

Nitric oxide (NO) is a potent effector molecule biosynthesised from L-arginine
by most cells. It participates in many biological functions, including non-
specific resistance to infections by bacteria, parasites and viruses. A high
output NO synthase (NOS2) regulated at the transcriptional level by cytokines
and bacterial products, is involved in natural resistance. Recently, NOS2 has
been identified in many types of cells, but NO synthase activity in human
macrophages/monocytes has long been questioned. Recent developments in
this field are discussed in this brief review.

Introduction

Evidence for the production of nitrite and nitrate by activated murine
macrophages [1] greatly facilitated the demonstration some ten years ago of
the biosynthesis of nitric oxide (the gas NO) from L-arginine [2–4]. NO is a
versatile molecule involved in vasodilation and neurotransmission which is
also a potent effector of the cytotoxic activity of activated macrophages
[5, 6].

The conversion of L-arginine into NO is catalysed by three isoforms of
NO synthase, and involves the oxidation of one of two terminal nitrogens of
its guanidine group. The other reaction product is L-citrulline. Another substrate
is molecular oxygen, and NADPH and tetrahydrobiopterin are essential cofactors
[7]. An inducible NO synthase (NOS2) was demonstrated, purified and cloned
for the first time in murine macrophages [8, 9] and is still sometimes called
Mac-NOS. Unlike constitutive NO synthases (NOS1 and NOS3), which are
dependent on intracellular calcium levels, the expression of NOS2 is regulated
by the transcription of its gene in response to exogenous stimuli [5]. NOS2
is a homodimer which releases NO in the presence of non-limiting quantities
of L-arginine, tetrahydrobiopterin and heme. When L-arginine and/or
tetrahydrobiopterine are limiting, part of the enzyme in the monomeric form

then produces O_2^- which combines with the NO, thereby generating the peroxynitrite ion [10, 11]. This ion is often considered as the reactive and toxic form of NO, including in the anti-parasitic activity of macrophages [12]. Independently of peroxynitrite, other reactive species derived from NO appear in oxygenated medium and it is very hard to determine their exact chemical nature. For reasons of simplicity, the name NO will be used in this article, without implying that this is the precise chemical form actually involved.

Induction of NOS2

Interferon-γ(IFN-γ), tumour necrosis factor (TNF) and compounds of microbial origin, such as lipopolysaccharide (LPS), are the most frequent inducers of NOS2 transcription, particularly in macrophages (Table 1). NOS2 induction generally requires co-operation between the inducing agents and there is synergy between IFN-γ and endogenous TNF [13]. One reason for this co-operation derives from the existence in the promoter region of NOS2 of numerous potential regulation sites, notably binding motifs for IRF1 (interferon regulatory factor 1) and κB sequences [7, 26]. NO can inhibit the activation of NF-κB by stabilising I-κB [26] or by direct nitrosylation of cys 62 [28]. In turn, NO can regulates its own production by feedback [29].

Table 1. Stimuli reported to induce NOS2 expression in macrophages *in vitro*

Murine macrophages	Human macrophages
IFN-γ [8]	*M. avium* [17, 18]
TNF* [13]	*T. cruzi* [19]
MIF [14]	*L. major* [20]
LPS* [8]	Poly IC [21]
Glycosylphosphatidylinositol [15]	gp 120 [22]
Hypoxia* [16]	VIH [23]
	Tumour cells [24]
	IFN-α [25]

*In synergy with IFN-γ.

NO influences the expression of cytokines. It inhibits the induction of macrophage IL-1 and IL-12 [30, 31], which may represent a regulation loop. Cytokines which suppress NOS2 transcription include IL-13, IL-10, IL-4 and TGF-β [32–35].

Various types of cells express NOS2: epithelial cells, mesenchymal cells and myeloid cells, etc. Of cells participating in the immune response, macrophages and neutrophils express NOS2 in response to cytokine or an infection [36, 37], whereas induction of NOS2 by lymphocytes has not been formally demonstrated.

Anti-Tumour Cytotoxicity

In vitro studies showed that NO is an effector of the anti-tumour cytotoxicity of murine macrophages [2], thereby concluding a long series of investigations conducted with this experimental system. In fact, NO exerts a rapid anti-proliferative effect by inhibiting the activity of ribonucleotide reductase, the enzyme limiting DNA replication [38], and can exert toxicity by inhibiting mitochondrial respiration [39] and nicking DNA [40].

In vivo, marked NO-dependent tumoricidal activity was observed towards syngeneic and xenogeneic tumours in BCG-injected mice. Expression of NOS2 is inversely related to production of metastases in murine melanoma cells [41]. The expression of NO synthase has been associated with macrophages infiltrating tumours, in animals and man, but it is still unclear whether NO has an anti-or pro-tumour effect under these conditions [42].

Another controversial issue is whether NO favours or prevents apoptosis. It has been shown that exposure of cells (including macrophages) to NO favours the expression of p53 and death through apoptosis [43, 44]. Yet recent studies claim that NO inhibits Fas-induced apoptosis [45], possibly through S-nitrosation of a critical sulphhydryl of cysteine proteases of the caspase family [46, 47]. Interestingly, some authors suggest that by inhibiting Fas-mediated apoptosis of autoreactive lymphocytes, NO could promote development of autoimmune diseases or lymphoma cells [45].

Antimicrobial Cytotoxicity

Numerous pathogenic micro-organisms, particularly those that develop intracellularly, are sensitive to NO or S-nitrosothiols (Table 2). Yet there are

Table 2. NO: Effecor of antimicrobial activity of activated murine macrophages

Pathogens	References
Fungi	
Cryptococcus neoformans	[48]
Histoplasma capsulatum	[49]
Parasites	
Schistosoma manson	[50]
Leishmania major	[51, 52]
Leishmania enriettii	[53]
Leishmania donovani	[54]
Toxoplasma gondii	[55]
Trypanosoma musculi	[56]
Entamoeba histolytica	[57]
Naegleria fowleri	[58]
Bacteria	
Mycobacterium leprae	[59]
Mycobacterium tuberculosis	[17]
Mycobacterium bovis	[60]
Francisella tularensis	[61]
Legionella pneumophila	[62]
Listeria monocytogenes	[63]
Rickettsia prowazekii	[64]

apparent contradictions in findings on the effect of NO in non-specific resistance to infections. Most experimental *in vivo* data derive from evaluation of infection by bacteria or pathogenic parasites of animals treated with NO synthase inhibitors. Most studies indicate greater sensitivity to infection in the treated animals. However, others suggest that NO counters multiplication of lymphocytes and so plays an immunosuppressive role which indirectly favours growth of pathogenic micro-organisms [65, 66]. Data on animals genetically lacking NOS2 seem to confirm the first alternative. In two independent studies, it has been shown that NOS2-/- mice are more sensitive to infection by bacteria or pathogenic parasites [67, 68]. Moreover, NO or NO-derived species mediate inhibition of malaria parasite by hepatocytes and monocytes *in vitro* [69–71]. A study of 191 African children with or without malaria revealed that urine and plasma nitrite and nitrate, as well as immunoreactive NOS2 in leukocytes, were inversely related to disease severity, suggesting that suppression of NO synthesis in severe malaria (*e.g.* cerebral malaria) contributes to pathogenesis [72].

NO has also recently been implicated in the induction of viral replication [73]. In several experimental models, induction of NOS2 blocks replication in macrophages of several types of viruses: flavivirus [74], vaccinia virus [75, 76], herpes simplex I [77], ectromelia [75] and even a retrovirus: friend virus [78].

NO and Human Macrophages

The longstanding controversy surrounding this subject seems far from over. It was hoped that the conditions of NOS2 induction would be defined by using the molecular tools available for analysis of NOS2 expression in the human system. In fact, the development of human anti-NOS2 antibodies and access to specific sequences of cDNA [79] quickly led to the demonstration of the induction of NOS2 under certain experimental conditions, but the catalytic activity was often weak or undetectable [80, 81]. The existence of an endogenous inhibitor has been proposed but experimental confirmation is still lacking. The low-level production of tetrahydrobiopterin by human macrophages does not seem to limit activity [82].

NO synthesis by human macrophages has been demonstrated by several groups (Table 2), but its role has been widely debated. The conditions of induction of NOS2 by human macrophages are quite special. *In vitro* treatment with IFN-γ, alone or combined with other cytokines or LPS, does not induce NOS2. This suggests that the antimicrobial cytotoxicity of IFN-γ-activated human macrophages probably results from other effector mechanisms [83, 84]. NOS2 expression has been noted in blood mononuclear cells from patients with rheumatoid arthritis, Grave's disease and tuberculosis [85–87]. *In vitro*, expression of NOS2 was preceded by phagocytic ingestion of living micro-organisms: *Mycobacterium avium, Trypanosoma cruzi, Leishmania major* (Table 1). It has recently been shown that binding of CD23, the low-affinity IgE receptor, induces the expression of NOS2. Stimulation of monocytes by IL-4, which promotes expression of CD23, followed by ligation of an anti CD23 antibody or an IgE/anti-IgE complex, induces NOS2 mRNA, expression of NOS2 detectable by specific antibodies, and production of stable reaction products (see 88 for a review). It has also been reported that human macrophages stimulated under these conditions inhibit the *in vitro* development of *L. major* [20]. Binding of CD69, which like CD23 is a member of the type C lectins family, also induces NO production by human monocytes, which then become cytotoxic to tumour cells *in vitro* [85].

Despite the ongoing debate [90, 91, 88], NO production by human monocytes is therefore a reality. However, in contrast to the murine system, the best studied to date, the inducing mechanisms are different and NO production is weaker. It has been proposed that the pressure of evolution may have resulted in restricted expression of NOS2 by these macrophages [91]. The suggestion is that NO is superfluous in antimicrobial cytotoxicity and is potentially toxic at high doses. NO would therefore be useless from a teleonomic point of view and its high output biosynthesis would be destined to disappear. Yet the between-species difference in induction of NOS2 by macrophages does not seem to depend on an evolutionary process alone. Indeed, macrophages of rabbit, cattle and deer also fail to respond to IFN-γ in the induction of NOS2 [84, 92, 93]. Other stimuli or signalling pathways are likely involved. Another more rational explanation of the between-species differences emerges from analysis of the NOS2-promoting regions. Two studies have revealed that specific sequences able to regulate ranscription of the NOS2 gene are different in mice and humans. Using the U937 monocyte cell line as a model of human macrophages, clear differences in the regulatory sequences of the promoter have been seen, notably the absence of the essential κB sequence in the mouse [94]. Another study using human liver epithelial cells has demonstrated the existence of multiple putative regulatory sequences up to 16 kb upstream of the initiation site [95]. These findings suggest that regulation of the transcriptional activity of NOS2 is both different and more complex in man, particularly in macrophages.

NO: Modulator of gene expression

In prokaryotes, NO or its derivatives activate the factors of genetic regulation SoxRS and OxyR, each of which controls a regulon of genes involved in defence against oxidative stress [96]. In OxyR, S-nitrosylation of cysteine 199 may enables the protein to assume a conformation favourable to its H_2O_2 and RSNO transcriptional activity [97]. In eukaryotes, it is emerging that biological radicals are not only toxic but may also serve as messengers in a new type of intracellular signalling. Hence, reactive oxygen species activates the translocation of transcription factor NF-κB [98] whereas NO inhibits it, as we have seen. Another mammalian *trans*-regulator, iron regulatory protein 1 (IRP1), is also sensitive to NO or related species (Table 3). IRP1 is an

Table 3.   NO: Modulator of gene expression

Trans-regulator	Submolecular target	Effect
Bacteria		
SoxR	2Fe-2S center	activation [99]
OxyR	cys 199	activation [97]
Yeast		
Lac9	Zn-thiolate	inhibition [100]
Mammals		
NF-κB	Cys 62	inhibition [28]
AP1	?	activation [101]
IRP1	4Fe-4S center	activation [102, 103]

[Fe-S] cluster protein which modulates intracellular iron concentration through co-ordinated post-transcriptional regulation of ferritin and transferrin receptor. It is bifunctional since it also possesses aconitase activity (citrate $\Rightarrow$ isocitrate). In response to modulation of the iron concentration, IRP1 switches from its aconitase function to its trans-regulatory function by binding to mRNA stem loops (iron responsive elements or IREs) located at 5' in ferritin, in the erythroid-specific form of 5-amino-levulinate synthase and in mitochondrial aconitase, and at 3' in the transferrin receptor. The structure of IRP1 is not yet known, but on the basis of the structure of crystallised mitochondrial aconitase, whose primary sequence around the [Fe-S] cluster is similar to that of cytosolic IRP1/aconitase, it is agreed that the [Fe-S] cluster and the substrate create a "bridge" between the different domains. Extrusion of the [Fe-S] cluster leads to opening of the protein, thereby rendering its IRE-binding domain accessible [104–106]. The dynamics of the [Fe-S] cluster of IRP1 are therefore a key feature which allows the protein to adapt to a particular environment and to respond to a change in activity. IRP1 is both the detector of cellular redox signals and the transducer of these signals to the mRNA.

Activation of NOS2 in various types of cells rapidly induces the conversion of IRP1 from its aconitase form to its regulatory, IRE-binding form [102]. Other groups have confirmed these results and have shown that, in response to this change in activity, the synthesis of ferritin is inhibited and the expression of the transferrin receptor is increased under certain conditions [103, 107, 108].

In conclusion, reactions between biological radicals (NO, O_2^-) and redox sites (transition metals, thiols) at critical catalytic or allosteric sites of essential proteins (enzymes, trans-regulators, ion channels, G-proteins) open up many alternative biochemical transduction pathways.

References

1. Stuehr D.J., Marletta M.A. Mammalian nitrate biosynthesis: mouse macrophages

produce nitrite and nitrate in response to *Escherichia coli lipopolysaccharide*. *Proc. Natal. Acad. Sci. USA*, 1985, **82:** 7738–7742.

2. Hibbs J.R. J.B., Taintor R.R., Vavrin Z. Macrophage cytotoxicity: role for L. arginine deiminase and imino nitrogen oxidation to nitrite. *Science*, 1987, **235:** 473–476.

3. Palmer R.M., Ferrige A.G., Moncada A. Nitric oxide release accounts for the biological activity of endothelium-derived relaxing factor. *Nature*, 1987, **327:** 524–526.

4. Ignarro L.J., Buga G.M., Wood K.S., Byrns R.E., Chaudhuri G. Endothelium-derived relaxing factor produced and released from artery and vein is nitric oxide. *Proc. Natl. Acad. Sci. USA*, 1987, **84:** 9265–9269.

5. Nathan C., Hibbs J.B. Jr. role of nitric oxide synthesis in macrophage antimicrobial activity. *Curr. Opin. Immunol.* 1991, **3:** 65–70.

6. Mc Micking, J, Xie Q and Nathan, C. Nitric oxide and macrophage function *Annu Rev. Immunol.* 1997, **15:** 323–350.

7. Nathan C., XIE Q.W. Nitric oxide synthases: roles, tolls and controls. *Cell,* 1994, **78:** 915–918.

8. Stuehr D.J., Marletta M.A. Induction of nitrite/nitrate synthesis in murine macrophages by BCG infection, lymphokines, or interferon-gamma. *J. Immunol.,* 1987, **139:** 518–525.

9. Lyons C.R., Orloff G.J., Cunningham J.M. Molecular cloning and functional expression of an inducible nitric oxide synthase from a murine macrophage cell line. *J. Biol. Chem.,* 1992, **267:** 6370–6374.

10. Xia Y., Zweier J.L., Proc. Natl. Acad. Sci. USA 1997, 94, 6954–6958. Superoxide and peroxynitrite generation from inducible nitric oxide synthase in macrophages.

11. Mayer B., Hemmens B. Biosynthesis and action of nitric oxide in mammalian cells. *Trends Biochem.* 197, **22:** 477–481.

12. Denicola A., Rubbo H., Rodriguez D., Radi R. Peroxynitrite-mediated cytotoxicity to *Trypanosoma cruzi*. *Arch. Biochem. Biophys.,* 1993, **304:** 279–286.

13. Drapier J.C., Wietzerbin J., Hibbs Jr. J.B. Interferon-gamma and tumor necrosis factor induce the L-arginine-dependent cytotoxic effector mechanism in murine macrophages. *Eur. J. Immunol.,* 1988, **18:** 1587–1592.

14. Cunha F.Q., Weiser W.Y., David J.R., Moss D.W., Moncada S., Liew F.Y. Recombinant migration inhibitory factor induces nitric oxide synthase in murine macrophages. *J. Immunol.,* 1993, **150:** 1908–1912.

15. Tachado S.D., Gerold P., Mcconville M.J., Baldwin T., Quilici D., Schwarz R.T., Schofield L. Glycosylphosphatidylinositol toxin of Plasmodium induces nitric oxide synthase expression in macrophages and vascular endothelial cells by a protein tyrosine kinase-dependent and protein kinase C-dependent signaling pathway. *J. Immunol.,* 1996, **156:** 1897–1907.

16. Melillo G., Musso T., Sica A., Taylor S.N., Cox G.W., Varesio L. A hypoxia-responsive element mediates a novel pathway of activation of the inducible nitric oxide synthase promoter. *J. Exp. Med.,* 1995, **182:** 1683–1693.

17. Denis M. tumor necrosis factor and granulocyte macrophage-colony stimulating factor stimulate human macrophages to restrict growth of virulent *Mycobacterium avium* and to kill avirulent *M. avium:* killing effector mechanism depends on the generation of reactive nitrogen intermediates. *J. Leuk. Biol.,* 1991, **49:** 380–387.

18. Dumarey C.H., Labrousse V., Rastogi N., Vargaftig B.B., Bachelet M. Selective mycobacterium avium-induced production of nitric oxide by human monocyte-derived macrophages. *J. Leukoc. Biol.,* 1994, **56:** 36–40.

19. Munoz-Fernandez M.A., Fernandez M.A., Fresno M. Activation of human

macrophages for the killing of intracellular *Trypanosoma cruzi* by TNF-a and IFN-g through a nitric oxide-dependent mechanism. *Immunol. Lett.,* 1992, **33:** 35–40.

20. Vouldoukis I., Riveros-Moreno V., Dugas B., Ouaaz F., Debre P., Moncada S., Mossalayi D.M. The killing of *Leishmania major by* human macrophages is mediated by nitric oxide induced after ligation of the FceRII/CD23 surface antigen. *Proc. Natl. Acad. Sci. USA,* 1995, **92:** 7804–7808.

21. Snell, J.C., Chernyshev, O., Gilbert, D.L., Colton, C.A., Polynucleotide induce nitric oxide production by human monocyte-derived macrophages. *J. Leukoc. Biol.,* 1997, **62:** 369–373.

22. Pietraforte D., Tritarelli E., Testa U., Minetti M. gp 120 HIV envelope glycoprotein increases the production of nitric oxide in human monocyte-derived macrophages. *J. Leukoc. Biol.,* 1994, **55:** 175–182.

23. Bukrinsky M.I., Nottet H.S.L.M., Schimidtmayerova H., Dubrovsky L., Flanagan C.R., Mullins M.E., Lipton S.A., Gendeleman H.E. Regulation of nitric oxide synthase activity in human immunodeficiency virus type 1 (VIH-1)-infected monocytes: Implications for HIV-associated neurological disease. *J. Exp. Med.,* 1995, **191:** 735–745.

24. Zembala M., Siedlar M., Marcinkiewicz J., Pryjma J., Human monocytes are stimulated for nitric oxide release in vitro by some tumor cells but not by cytokines and lipopolysaccharide. *Eur J. Immunol.,* 1994, **24:** 435–439.

25. Sharara A.I., Perkins D.J., Misukonis M.A., Chan S.U., Dominitz J.A., Weinberg J.B. Interferon (IFN)-alpha activation of human blood mononuclear cells in vitro and in vivo for nitric oxide synthase (NOS) type 2 mRNA and protein expression: possible relationship of induced NOS2 to the anti-hepatitis C effects of IFN-alpha in vivo. *J. Exp. Med.* 1997, **186:** 1495–1502.

26. Xie Q., A novel lipopolysaccharide-response element contributes to induction of nitric oxide synthase. *J. Biol. Chem.* 1997, **272:** 14867–14872.

27. Peng H.B., Libby P., Liao J.K. Induction and stabilization of I kappa B alpha by nitric oxide mediates inhibition of NF-kappa B. *J. Biol Chem* 1995, 270, **23:** 14214–14219.

28. Matthews J.R., Botting C.H., Panico M., Morris H.R., Hay R.T. Inhibition of NF-kappaB DNA binding by nitric oxide. *Nucleic Acids Res* 1996, **24:** 2236–2242.

29. Togashi H., Sasaki M., Frohman E., Taira E., Ratan R.R., Dawson T.M., Dawson V.L. Neuronal (type I) nitric oxide synthase regulates nuclear factor kappaB activity and immunologic (type II) nitric oxide synthase expression. *Proc. Natal. Acad. Sci. USA* 1997, **94:** 2676–2680.

30. Chujor C.S., Klein L., Lam C. Selective inhibition of interleukin-1 beta gene expression in activated RAW 264.7 macrophages by interferon-gamma. *Eur. J. Immunol.* 1996, **26:** 1253–1259.

31. Roth H., Hartmann B., Geerlings P., Kolb H. Interleukin-12 gene expression of macropaohages is regulated by nitric oxide. *Biochem. Biophys. Res. Commun.,* 1996, **224:** 159–163.

32. Bogdan C., Thuring H., Dlaska M., Rollinghoff M., Weiss G. Mechanism of suppression of macrophage nitric oxide release by IL-13: influence of the macrophage population. *J. Immunol.* 1997, **159:** 4506–4513.

33. Bogdan C., Vodovotz Y., Paik J., Xie Q.W., Nathan C. Mechanism of suppression of nitric oxide synthase expression by inerleukin-4 in primary mouse macrophages. *J. Leukoc. Biol.* 1994, **55:** 227–233.

34. Vodovotz Y., Bogdan C., Paik J., Xie Q.W., Nathan C. Mechanisms of suppression of macrophage nitric oxide release by transforming growth factor beta. J. Exp. Med. 1993, **178:** 605–613.

35. Bogdan C., Vodovotz Y., Paik J., Xie Q.W., Nathan C. Mechanism of suppression of nitric oxide synthase expression by interleukin-4 in primary mouse macrophages. *J. Leukoc. Biol.* 1994, **55**: 227–233.

36. Wheeler M.A,. Smith S.D., Garcia-Cardena G., Nathan C.F., Weiss R.M., Sessa W.C. Bacterial infection induces nitric oxide synthase in human neutrophils. *J. Clin. Invest.* 1997, **99**: 110–116.

37. Evans, T.J., Buttery L.D.K., Carpenter, A., Springall, D.R., Polak, synthase that prodiuces niration of ingested bacteria. *Proc. Natal. Acad. Sc. USA*, 1996, **93**: 9553–9558.

38. Lepoivre M., Fieschi F., Coves J., Thelander L., Fontecave M. Inactivation of ribonucleotide reductase by nitric oxide. *Biochem. Biophys. Res. Commun.*, 1991, **179**: 442–448.

39. Drapier J.C., Hibbs J.R. J.B. Differentiation of murine macrophages to express nonspecific cytotoxicity for tumor cells results in L-arginine-dependent inhibition of mitochondrial iron-sulfur enzymes in the macrophage effector cells. *J. Immunol.*, 1988, **140**: 2829–2838.

40. Nguyen T., Brunson D., Crespi C.L., Penman B.W., Wishnok J.S., Tannenbaum S.R. DNA damage and mutation in human cells exposed to nitric oxide in vitro. *Proc. Natl. Acad. Sci. USA.* 19, **89**: 3030–3034.

41. Dong, Z. Taroselsky, A.H., Q.I., X Xie, K., Fidler, I.J., Inverse correlation between expression of inducible nitric oxide synthase activity and production of metastasis in K-1735 murine melanoma cells. *Cancer Res.*, 1994, **54**: 789–793.

42. Jenkins D.C., Charles I.G., Thomsen, L.L., Moss D.W., Holmes L.S., Baylis S.A., Rhodes P., Westmore K., Emson P.C., Moncada S. Roles of nitric oxide in tumor growth. *Proc. Natl. Acad. Sci. USA*, 1995, **92**: 4392–4396.

43. Messmer U.K., Ankarcrona M., Nicotera P., Brune B. p53 expression in nitric oxide-induced apoptosis. *FEBS Lett.*, 1994, **355**: 23–26.

44. Forrester K., Ambs S., Lupold S.E., Kapust R.B., Spillare E.A. Weinberg W.C., Felley-Bosco E., Wang X.W., Geller D.A., Tzeng E., Billiar T.R., Harris C.C. Nitric oxide-induced p 53. accumulation and regulation of inducible nitric oxide synthase expression by wild-type p 53. *Proc. Natl. Acad. Sci. USA* 1996, **93**: 2442–2447.

45. Mannick J.B., Miao X.Q., Stamler J.S. Nitric oxide inhibits Fas-induced apoptosis. *J. Biol. Chem.* 1997, **272**: 24125–24128.

46. Mohr S., Zech B., Lapetina E.G., Brune B. Inhibition of caspase-3 by S-nitrosation and oxidation caused by nitric oxide. *Biochem. Biophys. Res. Commun.* 1997, **238**: 387–391.

47. Li J., Billiar T.R., Talanian R.V., K.I.M Y.M. Nitric oxide reversibly inhibits seven members of the caspase family via S-nitrosylation. Biochem. Biophys. Res. Commun. 1997, **240**: 419–424.

48. Alspaugh J.A., Granger D.L. Inhibition of Cryptococcus neoformans replication by nitrogen oxides supports the role of theses molecules as effectors of macrophage-mediated cytostasis. *Infect. Immun.*, 1991, **59**: 2291–2296.

49. Nakamura L.T., WU-Hsieh B.A., Howard D.H. Recombinant murine gamma interferon stimulates macrophages of the RAW cell line to inhibit intracellular growth of *Histoplasma capsuatum. Infect. Immun.*,1994, **62**: 680–684.

50. James S.L. Glaven J. Macrophage cytotoxicity against schistosomula of *Schistosoma mansoni* involve arginine-dependent production of reactive nitrogen intermediates. *J. Immunol.*, 1995, **143**: 4208–4812.

51. Green S.J., Nacy C.A. Antimicrobial and immunopathologic effects of cytokine-induced nitric oxide synthesis. *Current Opinion Infect. Dis.*, 1993, **6**: 384–396.

52. Liew F.Y., Millott S., Parkinson C., Palmer R.M.J., Moncada S. Macrophage killing of Leishmania parasite *in vitro* is mediated by NO from L-arginine. *J. Immunol.*, 1990, **144:** 4707–4794.

53. Mauel J., Corradin S.B., Buchmuller-Rouiller Y. Nitrogen and oxygen metabolites and the killing of Leishmania by activated murine macrophages. *Res. Immunol.*, 1991, **142:** 557–580.

54. Roach T.I., Kiderlen A.F., Blackwell J.M. Role of inorganic nitrogen oxides and tumor necrosis factor alpha in killing *Leishmania donovani* amastigotes in gamma interferon-lipopolysaccharide-activated macrophages from Lshs and Lshr congenic mouse strains. *Infect. Immun.*, 1991, **59:** 3935–3944.

55. Adams L.B., Hibbs J.R. J.B., Taintor R.E., Krahenbuhl J.L. Microbiostatic effect of murine-activated macrophages for *Toxoplasma gondii:* Role for synthesis of inorganic nitrogen oxides from L-arginine. *J. Immunol.*, 1990, **144:** 2725–2729.

56. Vincendeau P., Daulouede S. Macrophage cytostatic effect of *Trypanosoma musculii* involves and L-arginine-dependent mechanism. *J. Immunol.*, 1991, **146:** 4338–4343.

57. Lin J.Y., Chadee K. Macrophage cytotoxicity against *Entamoeba histolytica trophozoites* is mediated by nitride oxide from L-arginine. *J. Immunol.*, 1992, **148:** 3999–4005.

58. Fischer-Stenger K., Marciano-Cabral F. The arginine-dependent cytolytic mechanism plays a role in destruction of *Naegleria fowleri amoebae* by activated macrophage. *Infect. Immun.*, 1992, **60:** 5126–5131.

59. Adams L.B., Franzblau S.G., Vavrin Z., Hibbs Jr. J.B., Krahenbuhl, J.L. L-arginine-dependent macrophage effector functions inhibit metabolic activity of *Mycobacterium leprae. J. Immunol.*, 1991, **147:** 1642–1646.

60. Flesch I.E., Kaufmann, S.H. Mechanisms involved in mycobacterial growth inhibition by gamma a interferon-activated bone marrow macrophages: role of reactive nitrogen intermediates. *Infect, Immun.*, 1991, **59:** 3213–3218.

61. Fortier A.H., Polsinelli T., Green S.J., Nacy C.A. Activation of macrophages for destruction of *Francisella tularensis:* identification of cytokines, effector cells and effector molecules. *Infect. Immun.*, 1992, **60:** 817–825.

62. Summersgill J.T., Powel L.A., Buster B.L., Miller R.D., Ramirez J.A. Killing of *Legionella pneumophila* by nitric oxide in gamma-interferon-activated macrophages. *J. Leukoc. Biol.*, 1992, **52:** 625–629.

63. Beckerman K.P., Rogers H.W., Corbett J.A., Schreiber R.D., Mcdaniel M.L., Unanue E.R. Release of nitric oxide during the T-cell independent pathway of macrophage activation: its role in resistance to *Listeria monocytogenes. J. Immunol.* 1993, **150:** 888–895.

64. Turco J., Winkler H.H. Relationship of tumor necrosis factor alpha, the nitric oxide synthase pathway and lipopolysaccharide to the killing of gamma interferon-treated macrophage-like RAW 264.7 cells *by Rickettsia prowazekii. Infect. Immun.*, 1994, **62:** 2568–2574.

65. Albina J.E., Abate J.A., Henry J.R. W.L. Nitric oxide production is required for murine resident peritoneal macrophages to suppress mitogen-stimulated T cell proliferation. *J. Immunol.*, 1991, **147:** 144–148.

66. Langrehr J.M., Dull K.E., Ochoa J.B., Billiar T.R., ILdstad S.T., Schraut W.H., Simmons R.L., Hoffman R.A. Evidence that nitric oxide production by *in vivo* allosensitized cells inhibits the development of allospecific CTL. *Transplantation,* 1992, **53:** 532–640.

67. McMicking J.D., Nathan C., Hom G., Chartrain N., Fletcher D.S., Trumbauer M., Stevens K., Xie Q.W., Sokol K., Hutchinson N. Altered responses to bacterial

infection and endotoxic shock in mice lacking inducible nitric oxide synthase. *Cell,* 1995, **81:** 641–650.

68. Wei X.Q., Charles I.G., Smith A., Ure J., Feng G.J., Huang F.P., XU D., Muller W., Moncada S., Liew F.Y. Altered immune responses in mice lacking inducible nitric oxide synthase. *Nature,* 1995, **375:** 408-411.

69. Nüssler A., Drapier J.C., Renia L., Pied S., Miltgen F., Gentilini M., Mazier D. L-arginine-dependent destruction of intrahepatic malaria parasites in response to tumor necrosis factor and/or interleukin 6 stimulation. *Eur. J. Immunol.* 1991, **21:** 227–230.

70. Mellouk S., Green S.J., Nacy C.A., Hoffman S.L. IFN-gamma inhibits development of Plasmodium berghei exoerythrocytic stages in hepatocytes by an L-arginine-dependent effector mechanism. *J. Immunol.* 1991, **146:** 3971–3976.

71. Gyan B., Troye-Blomberg M., Perlman P., Bjorkman A Human monocytes cultured with and without interferon-gamma inhibit Plasmodium falciparum parasite growth in vitro via secretion of reactive nitrogen intermediates. *Parasite. Immunol.* 1994, **16:** 371–375.

72. Anstey N.M., Weinberg J.B., Hassanali M.Y., Mwaikambo E.D., Manyenga D., Misukonis M.A., Arnelle D.R., Hollis D., Mcdonald M.I., Granger D.L. Nitric oxide in Tanzanian children with malaria: inverse relationship between malaria severity and nitric oxide production/nitric oxide synthase type 2 expression. *J. Exp. Med.* 1996, **184:** 557–567.

73. Mannick J.B. The antiviral role of nitric oxide, *Res. Immunol.,* 1995, **146:** 693–697.

74. Kreil T.R., EIBL M.M. Nitric oxide and viral infection: NO antiviral activity against a flavivirus *in vitro,* and evidence for contribution to pathogenesis in experimental infection *in vivo. Virology,* 1996, **219:** 304–306.

75. Karupiah G., Xie Q.W., Buller R.M., Nathan C., Duarte C., McMicking D.J. Inhibition of viral replication by interferon gamma-induced nitric oxide synthase. *Science,* 1993, **261:** 1445–1448.

76. Melkova Z., Eteban M. Interferon gamma severely inhibits DNA synthesis of vaccinia virus in a macrophage cell line. *Virology,* 1994, 198.

77. Croen K.D. Evidence for antiviral effect of nitric oxide. Inhibition of herpes simplex virus type I replication. *J. Clin. Invest.,* 1993, **91:** 2446–2452.

78. Akarid K., Sinet M., Desforges B., Gougerot-Pocidalo M.A. Inhibitory effect of nitric oxide on the replication of a murine rerovirus *in vitro* and *in vivo. J. Virol.,* 1995, **69:** 7001–7005.

79. Chartrain N.A., Geller D.A., Koty P.P., Sitrin N.F., Nussler A.K., Hoffman E.P., Billiar T.R., Hutchinson N.I., Mudgett J.S., Molecular cloning, structure; and chromosomal localization of the human inducible nitric oxide synthase gene, *j. Biol Chem.,* 1994: **269:** 6765–72.

80. Weinberg J.B., Misukonis M.A., Shami P.J., Mason S.N., Sauls W.A., Dittman W.A., Wood E.R., Smith G.K., Mcdonald B., Bachus K.E., Haney A.F., Granger D.L. Human mononuclear phagocyte inducible nitric oxide synthase (iNOS): analysis of iNOS mRNA, iNOS protein, biopterin and nitric oxide production by blood monocytes and peritoneal macrophages. *Blood,* 1995, **86:** 1184–1195.

81. Reiling N., Ulmer A.J., Duchrow M., Ernst M., Flad H.D., Hauschildt S. Nitric oxide synthase: mRNA expression of different isoforms in human monocytes/macrophages. *Eur. J. Immunol.,* 1994, **24:** 1941–1944.

82. Werner E.R., Werner-Fehlmayer G., Fuchs D., Hausen A., Reibnegger G., Yim J.J., Pfeiderer W., Wachter H. Tetrahydrobiopterin biosynthetic activities in human macrophages, fibroblasts, THP-1 and T24 cells: GTP-cyclohydrolase-1 is stimulated

by IFN-γ, pyruvyltetrahydropterin synthase and sepiapterin reductase are constitutively present. *J. Biol. Chem.,* 1990, **265:** 3119–3125.

83. Schneemann M., Schoedon G., Hofer S., Blau N., Guerrero L., Schaffner A. Nitric oxide synthase is not a constituent of the antimicrobial armature of human mononuclear phagocytes. *J. Infect. Dis.,* 1993, **167:** 1358–1363.

84. Cameron M.L., Granger D.L., Weinberg J.B., Koxumbo W.J., Koren H.W. Human alveolar and peritoneal macrophages mediated fungistasis independently of L-arginine oxidation to nitrite and nitrate. *Am. Rev. Respir. Dis.,*1990, **142:** 1313–1319.

85. S.T. Clair E.W., Wilkinson W.E., Lang T., Sanders L., Misukonis M.A., Gilkeson G.S., Pisetsky D.S., Granger D.I., Weinberg J.B. Increased expression of blood mononuclear cell nitric oxide synthase type 2 in rheumatoid arthritis patients. *J. Exp. Med.* 1996, **184:** 1173–1178:

86. Lopez-Moratalla N., Calleja A., Gonzalez A., Perez-Mediavilla L.A., Aymerich M.S., Burrel M.A., Santiago E. Inducible nitric oxide synthase in monocytes from patients Graves' disease. *Biochem. Biophys. Res. Commun.* 1996, **226:** 723–729.

87. Nicholson S., Bonecini-Almeida M DA G., Lapa E. Silva J.R., Nathan C., al. Inducible nitric oxide synthase in pulmonary alveolar macrophages from patients with tuberculosis. *J. Exp. Med.* 1996, **183:** 2293–2302.

88. Dugas B., Mossalayi D.M., Damais C., Kolb J.P. Nitric oxide production by human monocytes/macrophages. Evidence for a role of CD23. *Immunol. Today,* 1995, **5:** 574–580.

89. DE Maria R., Cifone M.G., Trotta R., Rippo M.R., Festuccina C., Santoni A., Testi R. Triggering of human monocyte activation through CD69, a member of the natural killer cell gene complex of signal transducing receptors. *J. Exp. Med.* 1994, **181:** 735–745.

90. Denis M. Human monocytes/macrophages: NO or no NO? *J. Leukoc. Biol.,* 1994, **55:** 682–684.

91. Albina J.E.—On the expression of nitric oxide synthase by human macrophages. Why not NO? *J. Leukoc. Biol.,* 1995, **58:** 643–649.

92. Adler H., Frech B., Thony M., Pfister H., Peterhans E., Jungi T.W. Inducible nitric oxide synthase in cattle. Differential cytokine regulation of nitric oxide synthase in bovine and murine macrophages. *J. Immunol.,* 1995, **154:** 4710–4718.

93. Cross M.L., Thomson A.J., Slobe L.J., Griffin J.F., Buchan G.S. Macrophage function in deer. *Veter. Immunol. Immunopathol.,* 1996, **49:** 359–373.

94. Zhang X., Laubach V.E., Alley E.W., Edwards K.A., Sherman P.A., Russell S.W., Murphy W.J. Transcriptional basis for hyporesponsiveness of the human inducible nitric oxide synthase gene to lipopolysaccharide/interferon-γ. *J. Leukoc. Biol.,* 1996, **59:** 575–585.

95. DE Vera M.E., Shapiro R.A., Nussler A.K., Mudgett J.S., Simmons R.L., Morris J.R. S.M., Billiar T., Geller D.A. Transcriptional regulation of human inducible nitric oxide synthase (NOS2) gene by cytokines: initial analysis of the human NOS2 promoter. *Proc. Natl. Acad. Sci. USA,* 1996, **93:** 1054–1059.

96. Demple B. Study of redox-regulated transcription factors in prokaryotes. *methods* 1997, **11:** 267–278.

97. Hausladen A., Privalle C.T., Keng T., Deangelo J., Stamler J.S. Nitrosative stress: activation of the transcription factor OxyR. *Cell.* 1996, **86:** 719–729.

98. Muller J.M., Rupec R.A., Baeuerle P.A. Study of gene regulation by NF-Kappa B and AP-1 in response to reactive oxygen intermediates. *Methods* 1997, **11:** 301–312.

99. Nunoshiba T., Derojas-Walker T., Wishnok J.S., Tannenbaum S.R., Demple B.

Activation by nitric oxide of an oxidative-stress response that defends Escherichia coli against activated macrophages. *Proc. Natl. Acad. Sci. USA* 1993, **90:** 9993–9997.

100. Kroncke K.D., Fehsel K., Schmidt T., Zenke F.T., Dasting I., Wesener J.R., Bettermann H., Breunig K.D., Kolb-Bachofen V. Nitric oxide destroys zinc-sulfur clusters inducing zinc release frommetallothionein and inhibition of the zinc finger-type yeast transcription activator LAC9. *Biochem. Biophys. Res. Commun.* 1994, **200:** 1105–1110.

101. Haby C., Lisovoski F., Aunis D., Zwiller J. Stimulation of the cyclic GMP pathway by NO induces expression of the immediate early genes c-fos and junB in PC12 cells. *J. Neurochem.* 1994, **62:** 496–501.

102. Drapier J.C., Hirling H., Wietzerbin J., Kaldy P., Kuhn L.C. Biosynthesis of nitric oxide activates iron regulatory factor in macrophages. *EMBO J* 1993, **12:** 3643–3649.

103. Weiss G., Goossen B., Doppler W., Fuchs D., Pantopoulos K., Werner-Felmayer G., Wachter H., Hentze M.W. Translational regulation via iron-responsive elements by the nitric oxide/NO-synthase pathway. *EMBO J.* 1993, **12:** 3651–3657.

104. Kuhn L.C. Molecular regulation of iron proteins. *Baillieres Clin. Haematol.* 1994, 7, 763–785.

105. Klausner R.D., Rouault T.A., Harford J.B. Regulating the fate of mRNA: the control of cellular iron metabolism.*Cell.* 1993, **72:** 19–28.

106. Paraskeva E., Hentze M.W. Iron-sulphur clusters as genetic regulatory switches: the bifunctional iron regulatory protein-1. *FEBS Lett* 1996, **389:** 40–43.

107. Oria R., Sanchez L., Houston T., Hentze M.W., Liew F.Y., Brock J.H. Effect of nitric oxide on expression of transferrin receptor and ferritin and on cellular iron metabolism in K562 Human erythroleukemia cells. *Blood* 1995, **85:** 2962–2966.

108. Pantopoulos K., Hentze M.W. Nitric oxide signaling to iron-regulatory protein: direct control of ferritin mRNA translation and transferrin receptor mRNA stability in transfected fibroblasts. *Proc. Natl. Acad. Sci. USA* 1995, **92:** 1267–1271.

Immunopharmacology: Strategies for immunotherapy
S.N. Upadhyay (Ed)

5. Leishmanicidal Capacity of Human Macrophages: Role of FceRII/CD23 surface antigen

M.D. Mossalayi, I. Vouldoukis, A. Faili, P. Vincendeau and D. Mazier

Laboratoire d'Hématologie Cellulaire et Moléculaire, Faculté de Pharmacie Paris V.,
Paris; Inserm U313, CHU Pitié-Salpêtrière, Paris; and Laboratoire de parasitologie,
Université Bordeaux II, Bordeaux, France

Summary

Following infections with various helminths, macrophages are essential in initiating specific or innate immune response. Some of these pathogens inhabit macrophages and initiate a complex response involving most immune cells, T lymphocytes in particular. During some helminth infections, elevate plasma levels of total non-parasite specific IgE, high expression of surface and/or soluble fragments of the low affinity receptor for IgE (FceRII/CD23) are observed. Meanwhile, involvement of these factors during host protection or disease progression remains unclear. In regard to recent data, we here discuss the role of IgE and CD23 during *in vitro* and *in vivo Leishmania* infection or following immune challenge with *Leishmania* antigens. *In vitro*, the ligation of CD23 by appropriate ligands induces the production of various pro-inflammatory mediators and promoted intracellular killing of *L. major, L. braziliensis,* and *L. infantum* in human monocyte-derived macrophages. This effect is similar to that obtained with interferon-γ (IFN-γ) and is shown to involve the activation of tumor necrosis factor-α (TNF-α) and nitric oxide (NO). *In vivo,* the detection of IgE, CD23 and various cytokines during cutaneous leishmaniasis (C.L.) led us to provide a model for an immune response that involves CD23 and/or IgE during active disease.

Introduction

Human immune response in leishmaniasis remains to be clarified [1, 2] and most actual notions raised from the experimental murine models. These data show the central role of antigen-specific Th1- and Th2-like cells in anti-leishmania immune reactions [2, 3]. The inability to control leishmaniasis has been correlated with the absence of IFN-γ production by parasite-specific

T lymphocytes [3]. Leishmanicidal activity is correlated with an enhancement of the functions of monocytes/macrophages, with possible implication of the nitric oxide synthase pathway [3]. The combination of IFN-γ and TNF-α induces NO production by these cells [4, 5]. More recently, *in vivo* report definitively showed that NO is the effector factor for *L. major* elimination by macrophages [6].

Using polymerase chain reaction on human peripheral blood cells, early study showed the abundance of Th1-like cytokines in localized C.L., while cytokines from Th2-like lymphocytes were predominant in chronic disease [1, 7]. We have observed high levels of plasma IgE in most immuno-reactive cases in localized cutaneous leishmaniasis [8]. This phenomenon may be due to the *in vivo* production of IL-4, the switch factor for IgE [9], also detected in these individuals. Early reports postulated that the presence of IL-4 is related to disease progression and chronicity [10]. Using IL-4 transgenic mice together with various *in vivo* reports, more recent data clearly reject this dogma as they showed that the presence of IL-4 is observed during early immune response and does not always correlated with disease progression [8, 11–13]. The role of other cytokines will be detailed later in this issue.

Helminths, IgE CD23

Data now accumulated showing the rapid *in vivo* expression of IL-4 and IL-13 during anit-microbial activity. These data may explain how parasites lead to IgE increase because these factors are able to promote IgE gene expression. Expression of CD23 mRNA expression is strongly induced by IFNγ, IL-4 or IL-13 on human cells through Janus kinase activation and Stat6 DNA binding activity [14]. In an early study [8], we showed *in vivo* expression of CD23 in infiltrating hemopoietic cells in skin lesions from patients infected by *L. braziliensis* before and after antimonial treatment, as well as in intradermo-reaction sites in disease-free individuals from the same endemic area. Direct correlation was observed between the intensity of anti-*Leishmania* immune response and *in situ* expression of FcεRII/CD23, leukocyte infiltration, and serum levels of TNF-α and IgE [8]. Of particular interest, human macrophages acquire surface CD23 expression once they are infected by *Leishmania, Toxoplasma, or Mycobacteria,* while no functional FcεRI was detected [13]. Recent in vitro and in vivo data suggested a regulatory role for CD23/IgE during various human physiopathological situations such as hemopoiesis, anti-tumoral defense, inflammation, allergy, microbicidal activity of macrophages and eosinophils, skin diseases, and HIV infection [14–17].

CD23/FcεRII Signaling

CD23b isomer, not detected in mice, is an activation antigen expressed by various human hemopoietic cells, tissular epithelial cells and represents the major low affinity receptor for IgE (FcεRII) [14]. In its membrane and soluble forms, CD23 has multiple ligands that enable this molecule to trigger various functions in human and murine cells. In contrast to CD23a signals, all observed CD23b-mediated functions are strictly dependent upon CD23 cross-linking [18, 19]. Therefore, relatively high density of surface CD23b is required for optimal signaling. We have analyzed intracellular events leading to the release of inflamatory mediators from CD23$^+$ human cells following their activation with IgE-IC (Immune Complex) or CD23-mAb [15, 20]. It is important to note that CD23-signaling in freshly isolated human monocytes/macrophages is strictly dependent upon the activation state of the cells as CD23 cross-linking in activated cells caused cell inactivation, exhaustion and/or death [17].

Incubation of CD23$^+$ monocytes/macrophages with IgE/Ag induced an accumulation of intracellular cGMP and cAMP [19] in agreement with the fact that cyclic nucleotides analogues directly stimulated TNF-α production by these cells. It seems unlikely that this effect was the consequence of prostaglandin production since CD23-mediated cAMP accumulation in these cells was not altered by the cyclo-oxygenase inhibitor, indomethacin [20]. In contrast to CD23a, cross-linking of CD23b on all other human cells had low if any effect on Ca^{++} influx and phosphoinositide (P1) pathway [15]. Intrcellular accumulation of cGMP was observed during the first minutes of CD23-ligation, reached maximal levels at 5–10 min and decreased thereafter.

A role for the nitric oxide (NO)-dependent pathway in the generation of cGMP was proposed in various cellular models [21]. NO is a short-lived biological mediator produced by nitrogen hydroxylation of L-arginine in diverse cell types and catalyzed by NO synthase (NOS). Type-II NOS (also designed as inducible NOS, iNOS) differs from type I & III NOS in that it is functionally calcium independent [21]. Authors have thus asked if NO is induced following CD23 ligation. IgE-IC or anti-CD23 mAb clearly induce NO generation in monocytes/macrophages [18], through their ability to promote the transcription of NOS-II gene. Activation of NOS-II is followed by the generation of cGMP and nitrites, end products of NO-pathway [21], by human CD23$^+$ monocytes/macrophages [18, 19], eosinophils [22], myeloid leukemia [15], epithelial cells [16] as well as rat macrophages [23]. Addition of N$_G$-monomethyl-L-arginine (L-NMMA), an inhibitor of the NOS pathway, prior to CD23 ligation resulted in a dramatic decrease in NO generation and CD23-induced cell functions. L-NMMA, however, could not completely inhibit cAMP accumulation which suggests that CD23-mediated cAMP increase implied other intracellular transduction mechanism(s) [15]. Above signals were obtained with cells treated with IgE-IC or with anti-CD23, 135 mAb [18]. No NO generation was observed using many other CD23-mAb, which indicates that this effect is dependent upon triggering of specific CD23 epitope(s) [14]. No such events were observed in preactivated macrophages neither with cells expressed non-functional or cleaved CD23 on their surface.

In a U937 cell variant, these transduction events are followed by the activation of NFκB transcription factor and the modulation of proto-oncogene expression [15]. CD23-ligation increased c-fos/c-jun and promoted the expression of cell maturation-associated proto-oncogenes junB and c-fms, during the first 24 hours. Both IL-4 and CD23-mAb down regulated the expression of c-myb [15]. TNF-α m RNA was detected as early as 6 hr post CD23-ligation. Addition of both inhibitors of cAMP (Rp-isomer) and NO (L-NMMA) abolished most if not all CD23-mediated signals in target cells [34], which point out the importance of NO and cyclic nucleotides in membrane CD23-signal transduction. Other member of c-type lectin family, CD69, was also shown to mediate NO induction in human monocytes [24].

Above findings however suffer from the absence of data that linked CD23 molecule to cAMP or NOS machinery. CD23 intracytoplasmic portion is short and do not contain kinase domain [14]. Our preliminary data suggest that CD23 could be associated with other molecule(s) involved in signal transduction. In addition to NO and peroxides, CD23-ligation induces the release of TNFα, IL-1, IL-6 by human macrophages and keratinocytes 16, 20].

NO, CD23 and Leishmania Infection

During infectous diseases, CD23 may be detected in human monocyte-derived macrophages or dendritic cells [25], eosinophils and platelets [26]. Linking CD23 to NO generation asked its function in anti-microbial machinery of human macrophages. NO have long been recognized as possessing anti-microbial properties as it have been used in the meat industry to prevent spoilage by bacteria [27]. Most animal studies that have taken dietary nitrate into account have shown that infection induces NO synthesis [28]. NO is now recognized as a cytostatic or cytotoxic factor for multiple infectious agents including *leishmania, Mycobacterium, Toxoplasma* and *Trypanosoma* {21, 29]. NO is even emerged as the effector factor mediator for most *Leishmania* strains [3]. These data asked if NO is implied in CD23-mediated parasite killing. In fact, NO generation from human macrophages and the role of NO during infections in human is a mater of conflicting debate for several years.

In vitro, we have clearly shown that CD23-ligation mediates intracellular killing of *L. major, L. infantum* and *L. braziliensis* by human macrophages [18, 25]. The role of NO was clearly evidenced through the ability of NO inhibitors to completely abolish parasite killing, while chemical NO donors partially mimicked CD23-stimulation [25]. These data represented the first convincing evidence of the role of NO and CD23 in anti-microbial activities of human macrophages. In recent experiments, CD23-ligation permitted intracellular elimination of *M. avium* and *T. gondii* through NO-and TNF-α-dependent pathway (unpublished data). Therefore, IgE or antigen specific T cells may ligate CD23, induce macrophages bactericidal activity and therefore potentiate IFN-γ dependent NO generation [25].

Correlation Between *in vivo* and *in vitro* Data in CL

In vivo observations during CL (table 1) [7, 8, 30], although restricted to an endemic area in Brazil, showed a good relationship beween *in vivo* and *in vitro* cytokine expression and disease control. *In vitro*, two independent pathways may promote leishmanicidal activity of infected human macrophages: namely via IFN-γ receptor and CD23-ligation. IFN-γ and CD23/IgE induces TNF-α and NO production by infected human macrophages, a sequence involved in *L. major* killing by these cells [18]. However, TNF-α alone failed to directly induce *in vitro L. major* killing by macrophages.

When macrophages were stimulated with IFN-γ or CD23 alone, the addition of recombinant IL-4 or IL-10 dramatically reduces their leishmanicidal activity *in vitro* [18]. Of interest, macrophage activation through both CD23 and IFN-γ pathways protected them from inhibitory effect of IL-4 and/or IL-10 [18]. These data suggest that inhibitory cytokines can not eliminate effective leishmanicidal activity of human macrophages when both synergistic IFN-γ and CD23 pathways have been activated. This correlates exactly with *in vivo* cytokine patterns observed during effector immune responses before healing or during delayed type hypersensitivity (Figure). *In vitro*, in the absence of IFN-γ, the combination of IL-4, IgE immune complexes, TNF-α, and IL-10 failed to induce Leishmania clearance in infected human macrophages [25], correlating with *in vivo* expression of these factors [8] during disease exacerbation. Our *in vitro* data also correlated with study showing that anti-IL-10 restored the *in vitro* proliferation of peripheral blood T cells from infected patients [31]. Other important mediators were described for their potent role during *in vitro* Leishmania killing such as GM-CSF, M-CSF, TGF-β, IL-3, and IL-12 [1–3].

In contrast to most earlier studies, we suggest the involvement of L-arginine: NO pathway in Leishmania killing by human macrophages as: a) Addition of L-NMMA reversed leishmanicidal activity; (b) Protective effect of CD23 cross-linking correlated with NO generation; and (c) Chemical NO donors induces extracellular and intracellular killing of CL species. Furthermore, most NO inhibiting factors are known for their overexpression during disease progression [3]. In contrast to NOx, the generation of ROI has low or any role during the killing of *L. major* or *L. braziliensis* by human or murine macrophages [18, 32]. ROI inhibition by SOD and catalse even increased NO production by infected human macrophages [19]. This may be due to the interaction of NO with O_2^- which decreases the intracellular NO levels. This process may also result in the generation of peroxinitrites, potent toxic and pro-apoptotic agents [21]. Chronic exposure to peroxynitrites may also play a role in ulceration and disease progression. Meanwhile, these data do not exclude the role of peroxides in the killing of other Leishmania strains. Low levels of peroxides may also be required for the transcription of iNOS through their ability to activate NFκB transcription factor [33]. Therefore, parasite killing seems to imply a balanced network of multiple mediators shown in Fig. 1.

Implication for Treatment

In conclusion, these observations may explain the significance of IgE and

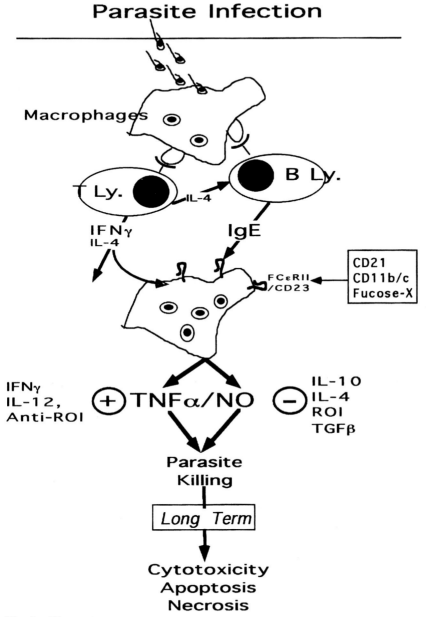

Fig. 1. **Human immune network following infection with *Leishmania* parasites.**

CD23 expression in CL, and various other protozoan infections. Data herein point out the importance of NO and its regulation in the anti-microbial activity of human macrophages and may indicate ways for better use of this pathway in the treatment of such diseases. Another therapeutic approach will be to directly ligate CD23 by synthetic ligands, and thus better targeting cellular responses and to prevent non-specific NOx-mediated toxicity. Arginine inhibitory analogues will be of interest to reverse the hypotension caused by cytokines in dogs [34] and sepsis in humans [35]; the question for many people is whether they will increase survival in each of these circumstances. Present technical limitations of such therapy include manipulating the timing of administration, selective inhibition of the inducible form of NOS, and the use of novel compounds that target endogenous NO generation. *In vivo* studies are now in progress to overcome these problems.

References

1. Modlin R.L. and Nutman T.B. 1993. Type 2 cytokines and negative regulation in human infections. *Curr. Opin. Immunol.* **5:** 511–117.
2. Reed .S.G. and Scott P. 1993. T-cell and cytokines responses in leishmaniasis. *Curr. Biology* **5:** 524–531.
3. Bogdan C., Gesser A., Solbach W. and Röööllinghoff M. 1996. Invasion, control and persistence of *Leishmania* parasites. *Curr. Opin. Immunol.* **8:** 517–525.
4. Green S.J., Nacy C.A. and Meltzer M.S. 1991. Cytoline-induced synthesis of nitrogen oxides in macrophages: a protective host response to leishmania and other intracellular pathogens. *J. Leuk. Biol.,* **50:** 93–103.
5. Liew F.Y., Millott S., Parkinson C., Palmer R.M.J. and Moncada S. 1990. Macrophage killing of *Leishmania* parasite *in vivo* is mediated by nitric oxide from L-arginine. *J. Immunol.* **144:** 4793–4802.
6. Stenger S., Thüüüring H., Röllinghoff M. and Bogdan C. 1994. Tissue expression of inducible nitric oxide synthase is closely associated with resistance of *Leishmania major. J. Exp. Med.* **180:** 783–793.
7. Primez C., Yamamura M., Uyemura K., Paes-Oliveira M., Conceicao-Silva F. and Modlin R.L. 1993. Cytokine patterns in the pathogenesis of human leishmaniasis. *J. Clin. Invest.* **91:** 1390–1395.
8. Vouldoukis I., Fourcade C., Paul-Eugène N., Arock M., Issaly F., Kolb J.P., da Silva O., Monjour L., Poinsot H., Dugas B., Debré P. and Mossalayi M.D. 1994. CD23 and IgE expression during human immune response to cutaneous leishmaniasis: Possible role in monocyte activation. *Res. Immunol.* **145:** 17–27.
9. Paul W.E. 1991. Interleukin-4: a prototypic immunoregulatory lymphokine. *Blood.* **77:** 1859–1870.
10. Reiner S.L. and Locksley R.M. 1995. The regulation of immunity to *Leishmania major. Annu. Rev. Immunol.* **13:** 151–177.
11. Coutinho S.G., Oliviera M.P., Da-Cruz A.M., De Luca P.M., Mendoça S., Bertho A.L., Soong L. and McMahon-Pratt D. 1996. T-cell responsiveness of american cutaneous leishmaniasis patients to purified *Leishmania pifanoi* antigens and *Leishmania braziliensis* promastigote antigens: Immunologic patterns associated with cure. *Exp. Parasitol.* **84:** 144–155.
12. Noben-Trauth N., Kropf P. and Müller I. 1996. Susceptibility of *Leishmania major* infection in interleukin-4-deficient mice. *Science* **217:** 987–990.
13. Scott P., Eaton A., Gause W.C., Zhou X.D. and Hondowicz B. 1996. Early IL-4 production does not predict susceptibility of *Leishmania major. Exp. Parasitol.* **84:** 178–187.
14. Mossalayi M.D., Arock, M. and Debré, P. 1997. CD23/FceRII: Signaling and clinical implication. *Int. Rev. Immunol.* **16:** 129–146.

15. Ouaaz F., Sola B., Issaly F., Kolb J.P., Davi F., Mentz F., Arock M., Paul-Eugène N., Körner M., Dugas B., Debré P. and Mossalayi M.D. 1994. Growth arrest and terminal differentiation of leukemic myelomonocytic cells induced through the ligation of CD23 antigen. *Blood.* **84:** 3095–3104.

16. Bécherel P.A., Mossalayi M.D., Ouaaz F., Le Goff L., Dugas B., Paul-Eugène N., Frances, C., Chosidow O., Kilcherr E., Guillosson J.J., Debré P. and Arock. M 1994. Involvement of the cAMP and nitric oxide pathway in the IgE-dependent activation of normal human keratinocytes. *J. Clin. Invest.* **93:** 2275–2279.

17. Ouaaz F., Ruscetti F.W., Dugas B., Mikovits J., Agut H., Debré P. and Mossalayi, M.D. 1996. Effects of IgE immune complexes on HIV-1 replication and cell death in infected U1 monocytes: Involvement of CD23/FceRII mediated nitric oxide and cyclic AMP pathways. *Mol. Med.* **2:** 38–49.

18. Vouldoukis I., Riveros-Moreno V., Dugas B., Ouaaz F., Bécherel P.-A., Moncada S. and Mossalayi M.D. 1995. The killing of Leishmania major by human macrophages is mediated by nitric oxide induced after ligation of the FceRII/CD23 surface antigen. *Proc. Natl. Acad. Sci. USA.* **92:** 7804–7808.

19. Dugas B., Mossalayi D.M., Damais C. and Kolb J.P. 1995. Nitric oxide production by human monocytes: evidence for a role of CD23. *Immunol. Today* **16:** 574–580.

20. Mossalayi M.D., Paul-Eugène N., Ouaaz F., Arock M., Kolb J.P., Kilchherr E., Debré P. and Dugas B. 1994. Involvement of FceRII/CD23 and L-arginine-dependent pathway in IgE-mediated stimulation of human monocyte functions. *Int. Immunol.* **6:** 931–934.

21. Moncada S. and Higgs E.A. 1993. The L-arginine-nitric oxide pathway. *N. Engl. J. Med.* **329:** 2002–2012.

22. Arock M., Le Goff L., Bécherel P.A., Dugas B., Debré P. and Mossalayi M.D. 1994. Involvement of FceRII/CD23 and L-arginine dependent pathway in IgE mediated activation of human eosinophils. *Biochem. Biophy. Res. Commun.* **203:** 265–271.

23. Alonso A., Carvalho J., Alonso-Torre S.R., Nunuz L., Bosca L. and Sanchez-Crespo M. 1995. Nitric oxide synthesis in rat teritoneal macrophages is induced by IgE/DNP complexes and cyclic AMP analogues, *J. Immunol.* **154:** 6475–6483.

24. De Maria R., Cifone M.G., Trotta R., Rippo M.R., Festuccia C., Santoni A., Testi R. 1994. Triggering of human monocyte activation through CD69, a member of the natural killer gene complex family of signal transducing receptors. *J. Exp. Med.* **180:** 1999–2004.

25. Vouldoukis I., Bé cherel P.-A., Riveros-Moreno V., Arock A., da Silva O., Debré P., Mazier D., and Mossalayi M.D. 1997. Interleukin-10 and interleukin-4 inhibit intracellular killing of *Leishmania infantum* and *Leishmania major* by human macrophages by decreasing nitric oxide generation. *Eur. J. Immunol.* **27:** 860–865.

26. Capron M. and Truong M.J. 1992. CD23 and eosinophils. *Res. Immunol.* **143:** 442–444.

27. Kerr R.H., Marsh C.N.T., Sheoeder W.F. and Boyer E.A. 1926. The use of sodium nitrite in the curing of meat. *J. of Agriculture Res.* **33:** 541–551.

28. Clark I.A. and Rockett K.A. 1996. Nitric oxide and parasitic diseases. *Adv. Parasitol.* **37:** 1–56.

29. Drapier J.C., Weitzerbin J. and Hibbs J.B. Jr. 1988. Interferon-γ and tumor necrosis factor induce the L-arginine-dependent cytotoxic effector mechanism in murine macrophages. *Eur. J. Immunol.* **18:** 1587–1590.

30. Barral-Netto M., Barral A., Brodskyn C., Carvalho E. M. and Reed S.G. 1995. Cytotoxicity in human mucosal and cutaneous leishmaniasis. *Parasite Immunol.* **17:** 21–28.

31. Carvalho E. M., Bacellar O., Brownell C., Regis T., Coffman R.L. and Reed S.G. 1994. Restoration of IFN-γ production and lymphocyte proliferation in visceral leishmaniasis. *J. Immunol.* **152:** 5949–5953.

32. Assreuy J., Cunha F.Q., Epperlein M., Noronha-Durta A., O'Donnell C.A., Liew F.Y., and Moncada S. 1994. production of nitric oxide and superoxide by activated macrophages and killing of *Leishmania major. Eur. J. Immunol.* **24:** 672–676.

33. Adcock I.M., Brown C.R., Kwon O. and Barnes P.J. 1994. Oxidative stress induces NFkB DNA binding and inducible NOS mRNA in human epithelial cells. *Biochem. Biophys. Res. Comm.* **199:** 1518–1524.

34. Kilbourn R.G., Owenschaub L.B., Cromeens D.M., Gross S.S., Flaherty M.J., Santee S.M., Alak A.M. and Griffith O.W. 1994. *N*-G-methyl-L-arginine, and inhibitor of nitric oxide formation, reverse IL-2-mediated hypotension in dogs. *J. Appli. Physiol.* **76:** 1130–1137.

35. Petros A., Lamb G., Leone A., Moncada S., Bennett D. and Vallance P. 1994. Effect of a nitric oxide synthase inhibitor in humans with septic shock. *Cardiovascular Res.* **28:** 34–39.

Immunopharmacology: Strategies for immunotherapy
S.N. Upadhyay (Ed)
Copyright © 1999 Narosa Publishing House, New Delhi, India

6. Maturation of Phagosome Containing Live Bacteria and Their Cross Talk with Endocytic Compartments

A. Mukhopadhyay

National Institute of Immunology, Aruna Asaf Ali Marg, New Delhi 110 067, India

Introduction

Phagocytosis is an important process in host defence and is mediated by complex receptor ligand interactions characterised by particle binding, internalisation and transport to the lysosomal or degradative compartments inside the cell [1]. Until recently it was thought that the nascent phagosome was destined to fuse with the lysosome to form a phagolysosome. But now it is clear that the process of phagosome maturation is much more complex and requires extensive remodulation of the phagosomal membrane [2, 3]. The phagosome maturation is also dependent on the intracellular signals triggered by the interaction of the specific receptor on the cell surface [4]. Several signalling molecules involved in phagocytosis have been identified and shown to differ depending on the specific receptor utilised during the phagocytosis. Moreover, phagosome maturation is now known to involve a variety of intracellular membrane fusion events with the early endosome and possibly with the Golgi or plasma membrane derived vesicles [1]. The dynamic exchange of phagosomal membrane with other intracellular vesicles is probably due to the delivery of hydrolytic enzymes and proton pumps to the matured phagosome [5]. Thus, the resultant phagosome with low pH and the hydrolytic enzymes becomes a hostile atmosphere for the invading microorganisms. However, many intracellular pathogens have evolved various strategies to ensure a safe life within the intravacuolar environment. These include:

(a) blocking of phagosome maturation into phagolysosome.
(b) inhibition of phagosome acidification.
(c) adapting to the acidic intravacuolar environment.
(d) lysing the vacuolar membrane to enter into the cytosol.

Micro-organisms and Their Fate in Phagocytes

Facultative intracellular pathogens have evolved multiple strategies to ensure intracellular survival. Thus, *Mycobacterium tuberculosis, Mycobacterium avium, Legionella peneumophilia, Salmonella typhimurium* and *Toxoplasma gondii* survive and proliferate in the vacuolar compartments that do not mature into phagosomes. Phagosomes containing *M. tuberculosis* express early endosomal markers, the transferrin receptor and also contains MHC class I and MHC class II molecules, indicating that phagosome maturation process is partially blocked in *M. tuberculosis* containing phagosome [6]. Recent reports have shown that such phagosomes have low levels of late endosomal/ lysosomal markers such as lysosomal glycoproteins so the later stages of the development of phagosomes containing *M. tuberculosis* are still not clear [7, 8]. However, the protozoans like *Trypanosoma cruzi* (9) and bacteria such as *Shigella flexneri* (10) and *Listeria monocytogenes* [11] reside transiently in the phagosomal compartments after entry into the cells. Subsequently, phagosomal membranes undergo pathogen-directed lysis and escape of the pathogen to the cytoplasm. In contrast, parasitophorous vacuoles that contain *Leishmania* species are rich in lysosomal glycoprotein and lysomal enzymes [12, 13]. Parasitophorous vacuoles containing *Leishmania mexicana* or *Leishmania donovani* do not express cation independent mannose 6 phosphate receptor (CI-M6PR) even two days after infection but another prelysosomal marker, rab7 is detected on this phagosome [14, 15]. Thus, *Leishmania* seem to reside in a phagosome like compartment and maturation of these phagosomes involves fusion with prelysosomal and lysosomal compartments. In the endocytic compartments, progressive acidification occurs reaching the pH values of 4.5 to 5 in secondary lysosomes, the optimal pH for activity of many hydrolases. This acidification is mediated through the expression of vacuolar ATPases and the proton pump on the phagosomal membrane. Some organisms prevent the expression of vacuolar ATPase and proton pump on the phagosomal membrane and therby they survive. The intravacuolar pH of the phagosome containing live *T. gondii* is neutral (pH 6.8-7) when the parasite enters into the macrophages through active endocytosis. In contrast, the phagosomes containing heat killed *T. gondii* or the antibody coated parasite rapidly reach the pH value close to 5 [16]. These results suggest that phagosome acidification depends on the route of entry used by the parasite. But certain pathogens survive even in the acidified phagosome such as *Coxiella burnetti* [17] and *Leishmania*[18]. So far, very little is known about the mechanism of adaptation of these organisms to this acidic environment.

Some pathogens appear to have developed mechanisms to modulate the redistribution of the endosomal and lysosomal marker molecules. *Salmonella typhimurium* containing phagosomes fuse with the compartment containing lysosomal glycoprotein (lgp), bypassing compartments containing cation-dependent mannose 6-phosphate receptor (CD-M6PR) or CI-M6PR which are normally encountered along the endocytic route. But there are conflicting report regarding the maturation of *Salmonella* containing phagosome. Recent studies have revealed [19] that *Salmonella* reside in a phagosome which is acidic (pH 4-5), contrary to the previous report that suggests a delay in phagosomal acidification [20]. A recent report has shown that *Salmonella* phagosome mediates rapid and complete fusion with lysosomes [21], another group reported the inihibition of *Salmonella* phagosome fusion with lysosomes [22]. Moreover, another possibility is that *Salmonella* phagosome fuse with a modified lysosome which lack vacuolar ATPase and proton pump and these two molecules are selectively eliminated from the mature phagolysosome. These results suggest that *Salmonella* may have the capacity to selectively fuse with vesicles carrying different markers in order to create a unique phagosomal environment that allow their survival.

Endocytosis Versus phagocytosis

Endocytosis and phagocytosis are the two primary mechanisms used by eukaryotic cells to internalise macromolecules from the extracellular milieu [23]. Endocytosis occurs in most eukaryotic cells and is essential for the uptake of nutrients and maintenance of cell homeostasis. Essentially, two types of endocytosis have been described: receptor mediated and fluid phase. Receptor mediated endocytosis involves the internalisation of the cell surface receptor through specific areas on the plasma membrane (coated pits, caveolae) and is highly efficient and selective. Fluid phase endocytosis is a relatively nonselective constitutive cellular process that is less completely understood. After internalization, endocytosed materials and receptor bound particles are delivered to a common endosomal compartment where they are sorted and targeted to other intracellular destinations including a putative recycling compartment, a trans-Golginetwork and diversion to lysosomal degradative compartments. Individual macromolecules or small particles (<100 nm) are usually internalised by endocytosis. In contrast to endocytosis, phagocytosis is a similar function of specialised cells such as macrophages for internalization of large particles (~ 500 nm), bacteria and other pathogens. After internalization, phagosome fuses with the degradative compartment and matures into phagolysosome [24]. Thus, while endocytosis and phagocytosis employ different mechanisms for internalization, the fate of internalised material is same. It has been shown that small GTP binding proteins regulates endocytosis in mammalian cells but the mechanism of vesicular transport containing the microorganisms in phagocytic pathway is not clearly documented. Moreover, it will be interesting to know how the live organisms modulate the central process of endocytosis for their survival in the hostile atmosphere of phagocytes. Different microorganisms mature into different kinds of compartments in respect to phagosomal composition, this may be due to the different kinds of crosstalk between the microorganism containing phagosome with the other intracellular compartment and their modulation by the live organisms.

Role of Small GTP Binding Proteins in Vesicular Transport

Membrane trafficking pathways mediate the movement of the membrane bound compartments between plasma membrane and defined intracellular compartments. During the past few years, it has been shown that GTP binding proteins are versatile molecular switches that are involved in vesicle budding and fusion of vacuolar structures in membrane trafficking event [25]. The small GTP binding proteins, whose members include the product of the ras, rab, rho, ran, ypt gene families, represent a large group of proteins involved in regulating numerous and diverse cellular functions including growth, differentiation and vesicular transport. All these proteins regulate membrane trafficking events by altering between two conformations in a nucleotide dependent fashion where GTP bound form turns the protein "on" and hyrolysis of the GTP to GDP turns the protein "off". These activities are regulated by a series of generic and compartment specific proteins. Small GTP binding protein homologues have been identified in many different species and conservation of their sequences suggests a similar function in different organisms. Several groups have shown that transport of materials from one intracellular compartment to another occurs through vesicle budding and fusion. Vesicles containing cargo bud from the donor compartment and deliver their contents to the acceptor compartment by fusion with the later. The processes of vesicle budding, docking and fusion with acceptor compartment are regulated by a series of generic and compartment specific proteins. Among them rab and ypt subfamilies are involved in regulating vesicular transport in mammalian cells and yeast, respectively. These proteins are specifically localised on distinct intracellular compartments and presumably control a specific transport step [26, 27].

Among the monomeric small GTPases, the rab family of ras related proteins [28] are well characterised as regulators of intracellular trafficking during endocytosis and secretion. Rab proteins are specifically localised to the cytoplasmic surface of the intracellular compartments that they subserve. Rab 1 and rab 2 are found to be localised in ER and cis-Golgi. Similarly, rab 6 and rab 9 are localised in medial Golgi and trans Golgi respectively [29, 30]. Rab 4, rab 5, rab 11, rab 18 and rab 24 have all been shown to be associated with early endocytic compartments, suggesting that the early endocytic compartment is highly complex with multiple function [31–33]. Internalised receptor and ligand first enter the peripheral sorting endosome where the membrane proteins destined for degradation or trans Golgi network (TGN) are sorted away from membrane proteins target for recycling back to plasma membrane. A substantial body of evidence indicates that rab 5 regulates endocytosis from the plasma membrane to the early endosomes and is also involved in homotypic fusion between the early endosomes [34]. Rab 4 appears to control the recycling from the early endosomes to the plasma membrane. Recent studies indicate that rab 11 regulates the recycling through the perinuclear endosomes. Rab 7 and rab 9, perhaps others to be identified, are associated with the late endosomal compartments. Rab 9 has been shown to regulate the traffick from the late endosome to TGN and rab 7 has been shown to regulate the traffick from the early to late endosomes/lysosome [35-37]. It has also been shown that ypt 7, the yeast homologue of mammalian rab 7 regulates the transport between the late endosome to the vacuole, a lysosome like compartment in yeast. Among the endocytic rabs, rab 5 has been most extensively studied. Rab 5 is active in GTP bound form and is regulated by multiple factors like N-ethylmaleimide sensitive fusion proteins (NSF), PI3 kinase, phosphlipase A2 etc [38-40]. Rab 5 and rab 7 both regulate endocytosis but rab 7 functions downstrean of rab 5. However, the exact relationship among all these factors in the overall mechanism of intracellular trafficking during endocytosis is largely unknown.

A current model (Fig. 1) suggests that rab proteins are predominantly found on cellular membranes but a significant fraction is also present in the cytosol as complex with guanine nucleotide dissociation inhibitor (GDI). GDI presents the complex to the specific organelles, this may be catalysed by GDI displacement factor (GDF) in conjunction with guanine nueotide exchange factor (GEF). GTP bound rab proteins are recruited onto nascent transport vesicles and catalyse the association of V SNARE (Soluble NSF attachment protein (SNAP) receptor on vesicle) with T SNARE (SNAP receptor on target) to accomplish the transport vesicle delivery. After the fusion, GTPase activating proteins (GAP) increase the GTPase rate of the rab protein, converting it into its GDP-bound conformation. Unoccupied GDI then retrieve the rab protein for another round of vesicular transport [41, 42]. This is a generalised model (Fig. 1) but most of the interacting proteins for a particular rab have not been identified.

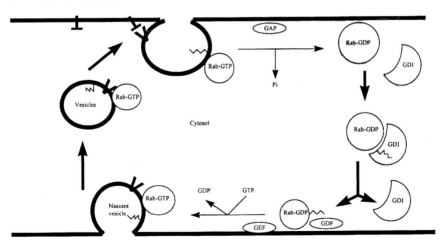

Fig. 1. Schematic representation of the membrane trafficking cycle.

The docking and the fusion of the vesicle is further regulated by a series of proteins. Rab proteins when bind to the nascent vesicles, somehow activate the V SNARE which in turn binds with respective T SNARE, then the vesicles dock with each other. But the fusion is mediated by other proteins like NSF and SNAP. SNAP proteins bind to the SNARE complex at the attachment site of the vesicles and its target. Each V SNARE and T SNARE complex binds between 3 to 6 SNAP proteins and then NSF binds to this complex. Subsequently NSF hydrolyses the ATP and uses the energy to disrupt the docking complex and releasing the SNAP protein [43, 44]. Although the precise role of different fusion proteins and their interaction with a particular rab in the mechanism of vesicular transport between different compartments is not clearly known.

Intracellular pathogens exploit the host cell function for their survival in the intracellular atmosphere. It will be interesting to evaluate whether intracellular pathogens like *Salmonella* alter the function of any of these proteins to avoid or induce the specific interactions of phagosome with other vacuolar compartments. Most of the knowledge of phagosome maturation is mainly based on the morphological observations. Lack of proper biochemical assays to monitor the phagosome maturation and their crosstalk with other endocytic compartments does not allow the dissection of the signal transduction mechanisms involved in this process. Promising experimental approaches to answer these questions inclued the isolation of intact vacuole containing intracellular pathogens and their interaction with other endocytic compartments using *in vitro* reconstitution assays and permeabilised cell systems.

Role of GTP Binding Proteins in Phagocytosis

Invading microorganisms modulate this central process for their survival in the phagocytic cells. The formation, function and the fate of phagosome maturation is also controlled by the fusion of different endocytic vesicles. Virtually all studies on the phagosome maturation have been carried out with model particles or dead microorganisms whose final fates appears to be similar to endocytic route and culminates with the fusion of lysosomes. Recently, it is possible to analyse the protein and lipid composition of the phagosome during their maturation using highly purified phagosomes at different times after internalisation. After a short period of internalisation, phagosome appears to be rich in certain membrane proteins such as transferrin receptor, mannose receptor and rab5, which subsequently decreases as phagosomes, matures. In contrast, other proteins like mannose 6 phosphate receptor, vacuolar ATPase, lamp molecules accumulate in the matured phagosome [45, 46]. Moreover, it has been shown that phagosomal trafficking inside the macrophages also depends on the size of the particle [47].

Transport of phagosomes containing different microorganisms in whole cells have been widely studied but little information has emerged on the mechanism of membrane recognition and the fusion between the phagosomes containing live organisms with the other intracellular vesicles. A major obstacle has been the difficulty in manipulating the cytosolic environment surrounding the intracellular vesicles. One approach to overcome this problem has been to reconstitute vesicle transport events in broken cell preparations. It has been shown that *in vitro* reconstitution of early phagosome containing model particles fusion with endosome requires cytosol, ATP and other fusion proteins like NSF (48). Thereby, it is possible that together with SNAPs, NSF plays a key role in interacting with respective SNAREs. Phagosome-endosome fusion is also sensitive to nonhydrolysable GTP analogue like GTPγS suggesting the role of small GTP binding proteins in the docking and fusion with respective compartments. Several lines of evidences have also indicate the role of heterotrimeric G proteins in the phagosome endosome fusion [49]. Recently it has been possible to reconstitute the endosome and phagosome fusion using live *Listeria* to understand how the live bacteria modulate the fusion process [50]. It has been shown that rab5 regulates the phagosome-endosome fusion and live organism can upregulate this fusion process by recruiting fusion proteins like rab5 and NSF. Similarly, phagosome lysosome fusion can also be reconstituted using permeabilised cell preparations [51]. The phagosome lysosome fusion is also requiring cytosol, NSF and rab proteins. Thus the reconstitution assay offer an advantage to determine the role of different signal transduction intermediates in phagocytosis of the life organisms. It will be interesting to determine how live organisms exploit the membrane fusion process inside the host cells to ensure safe life.

Perspectives

The extraordinary diversified strategies used by the different pathogens for their survival inside the hostile atmosphere of the phagocytes mainly mediates by the acquisition of the signals from the other intracellular compartments. The identification and characterisation of the complex mechanisms utilised by intracellular parasite to interfere with the normal process of phagosome maturation will be extremely important to understand the mechanism of their survival. Moreover, one common way the microroganisms proliferates inside the cells is by blocking the phagosome maturation and intravacuolar acidification. Further studies of membrane trafficking events in phagocytic pathway and their relationship with small GTP binding proteins would be necessary to fully understand how the live bacteria exploit the trafficking pathway to its own advantage and survive in host cells.

References

1. Beron, W., Alvarez-Dominguex, C., Mayorga, L., and Stahl, P. 1995. *Trends. Cell. Biol.* **5**: 100.
2. Desjardins, M., Huber, L.A., Parton, R.G., and Griffths, G. 1994a. *J. Cell. Biol.* **124**: 677.
3. Desjardins, M., Celis, J.E., van Meer, G., Dieplinger, H., Jahraus, A., Griffith, G. and Huber, L.A. 1994b. *J. Biol. Chem.* **269**: 32194.
4. Greenberg, S. 1995. *Trends. Cell. Biol.* **5**: 93.
5. Kornfield, S. and Mellman, I. 1989. *Annu. Rev. Cell. Biol.* **5**: 482.

6. Clemens, D.I. and Horwitz, M.A. 1995. *J. Exp. Med.* **181:** 257.
7. Sturgill-Koszycki, S. et. al., 1994. *Science* **263:** 678.
8. Xu, S. et. al., 1994. *J. Immunol.* **153:** 2568.
9. Hall, B.F. et. al., 1992. *J. Exp. Med.* **176:** 313.
10. High, N. et. al., 1992. *EMBO J.* **11:** 1991.
11. Portnoy, D.A., Jacks, P.S. an Hinrichs, D.J. 1988. *J. Exp. Med.* **167:** 1459.
12. Antoine, J.C. et. al., 1991. *Infect. Immun.* **59:** 764.
13. Russel, D.G., Xu, S.M. and Chakraborty, P. 1992. *J. Cell Sci.* **103:** 1193.
14. Lang, T. et. al., 1994. *J. Cell Sci.* **107:** 69.
15. Lang, T. et. al., 1994. *J. Cell Sci.* **107:** 2137.
16. Sibley, L.D. 1995. *Trends Cell Biol.* **5:** 129.
17. Maurin, M. et. al., 1992. *Infect. Immun.* **60:** 5013.
18. Antoine, J.c. et. al., 1990. *Infect. Immun.* **58:** 779.
19. Rathman, M., Sjaaastad, M.D. and Falkow, S 1996. *Infect. Immun.* **64:** 2765.
20. Alpuche-Aranda, C.M., swanson, J.A., Loomis, W.,P., and Miller, S.I. 1992. *Proc. Natl. Acad. Sci. USA.* **89:** 10079.
21. Ho, Y.K., Aranda, C., Berthiaume, E., Jinks, T., Miller, S.I. and Swanson, J.A. 1996. *Infect. Immun.* **64:** 3877.
22. Buchmeier, N.A. and Heffron, F. 1991. *Infect. Immun.* **59:** 2232.
23. Schwart, A.L. 1990. *Annu. Rev. Immunol.* **8:** 195.
24. Greenberg, S., Khoury, J.E., Virgili, F., Kaplan, E.M. and Silverstein, S.C. 1991. *J. Cell. Biol.* **113:** 757.
25. Blum, J.S., Diaz, R., Mayorga, L.S. and Stahl, P.D. 1993. 'Reconstitution of endosomal transport and proteolysis,' in *Subcellular Biochemistry*, **9:** 69–93, Ed. Bergeron, J.J.M. and Harris, J.R. Plenum press, New York.
26. Goud, B. and Mc Caffrey, M. 1991. *Curr. Opin. Cell Biol.* **3:** 626–633.
27. Rothman, J.E. 1994. *Nature* **372:** 55.
28. Valencia, A., Chardin, P., Wittinghofer, A. and Sander, C. 1991. *Biochem.* **30:** 4637.
29. Chavrier, P., Parton, R.G., Hauri, H.P., Simons, K. and Zerial, M. 1990. *Cell.* **62:** 317.
30. Goud, B., Zahraui, A., Tavitan, A. and Saraste, J. 1990. *Nature* **345:** 553.
31. Sluijs, V., Hull, P.M., Zahraoui, A., tavitan, A., Goud, B. and Mellman, I. 1991. *Proc. Natl. Acad. Sci. USA.* **88:** 6313.
32. Bucci, C., Parton, R.G., Mather, I.H., Stunnenberg, H., Simons, K., Hflack, B. an Zerial, M. 1992. *Cell.* **70:** 715.
33. Li, G. and Stahl, P.D. 1993. *J. Biol. Chem.* **268:** 24475.
34. Barbieri, M.A., Roberts, R.L., Mukhopadhyay, A. and Stahl, P.D. 1996. *Biocell.* **20:** 331.
35. Mukhopadhyay, A., Barbieri, A.M., Funato, K., Roberts, R. and Stahl, P.D. 1997. *J. Cell. Biol.* **136:** 1227.
36. Mukhopadhyay, A., Funato, K. and Stahl, P.D. 1997. *J. Biol. Chem.* **272:** 13055.
37. Lombardi, D., Soldati, T., Riederer, M.A., Goda, Y., Zerial, M. and Pfeffer, S. 1993. *EMBO J.* **12:** 677.
38. Diaz, R. L., Mayorga, L.S., Weideman, P.J., Rothman, J.E. and Stahl, P.D. 1989. *Nature* **339:** 398.
39. Mayorga, L.S., Clombo, M.I., Lennartz, M., Brown, E.J., Rahman, K.H., Weiss, R., Lennon, P.J. and stahl, P.D. 1993. *Proc. Natl. Acad. Sci. USA.* **90:** 20255.
40. Li. G., D'Suza-Schorey, C., Barbieri, M.A., Roberts, R.L., Klippel, A., Williams, L.T. and Stahl, P.D. 1995. *Proc. Natl. Acad. Sci. USA.* **92:** 10207.
41. Pfeffer, S. 1994. *Curr. Opin. Cell. Biol.* **6:** 522.

42. Rothman, J.E. and Wieland, F.T. 1996. *Science* **272:** 227.
43. Sollner, T., Whiteheart, S.W., Brunner, M., Erdjument-Bromage, H., Geromanos, S., Tempst, P. and Rothman, J.E. 1993. *Nature* **362:** 318.
44. Soggard, M., Tani, K., Ye, R.R., Geromanos, S., Tempst, P., Kirchhausen, T., Rothman, J.E. and Sollner, T. 1994, *Cell* **78:** 937.
45. Desjardins, M., Huber, L.A., Parton, R.G. and Griffiths, G. 1994. *J. Cell Biol.* **124:** 677.
46. Desjardins, M. et. al., 1994. *J. Biol. Chem.* **269:** 32194.
47. Berthiaume, E.P., Medina, C., and Swanson, J.A. 1995. *J. Cell. Biol.* **129:** 989.
48. Pitt A., Mayorga, L.S., Stahl, P.D. and Schwartz, A.L. 1992. *J. Clin. Invest.* **90:** 1978.
49. Beron, W., Colombo, M.I., Mayrga, L.S. and Stahl, P.D. 1996. *Arch. Biochem. Biophys.*
50. Alvarez-Dominguez, C., Barbieri, A.M., Beron, W., Wandinger-Ness, A and Stahl, P.D. 1996. *J. Biol. Chem.* **271:** 13834.
51. Funato, K., Beron, W., Yang, C.Z., Mukhopadhyay, A. and Stahl, P.D. 1997. *J. Biol. Chem.* **272:** 16147.

Immunopharmacology: Strategies for immunotherapy
S.N. Upadhyay (Ed)

7. Potentiation of Interleukin-2 Induced NK Activation by Simultaneous Exposure to Tumor Target Cells

S. Dhillon and R.K. Saxena

School of Life Sciences, Jawaharlal Nehru Uiversity, New Delhi 110067, India

Introduction

Natural killer (NK) cells and cytotoxic T cells (CTLs) constitute two types of lympocytes which can mediate direct lysis of target cells. CTLs have to be induced by antigens. Both NK cells and CTLs have been implicated in anti tumor immunosurveillance mechanisms. Interleukin-2 (IL-2), a cytokine which induces proliferation of sensitized T cells, can also augment cytotoxic activity of NK cells [1, 2, 3]. Nature of IL-2 receptors on NK cells is different from those on T lymphocytes. While IL-2 receptors on T cells comprise of three transmembrane protein chains, namely alpha, beta and gamma chains, IL-2 receptors on NK cells lack the alpha chain and as a consequence have significantly lower affintiy for IL-2 [4]. Relatively higher doses of IL-2 are therefore needed to activate NK cells.

CTLs recognize target cells through specific T cell receptors which recognize antigenic peptide associated with MHC molecule on the target cells [5]. NK cell receptors which participate in target cell recognition have not yet been clearly defined. NK cells express certain receptors which recognize target cell MHC molecules and send a negative signal to prevent the target lysis [6]. These receptors termed killer cell inhibitory receptors (KIRs) generally have ITIM motif on the cytoplasmic portions which mediate the negative signal [7]. Certain KIR like molecules having ITAM activating motif instead of the ITIM motif have recently been described [8]. Such ITAM bearing receptors may constitute good candidates for target recognition receptors on NK cells.

Since IL-2 receptor as well as the target recognition receptors on NK cells, can transduce activating signals, it was of interest to examine if these signals can have synergistic effect on NK cell activation. In the present study we have compared NK cell activation in response to (a) IL-2, (b) fixed tumor target and (c) both of these agents together. Our results indicate that fixed tumor target cell can significantly boost NK activation in response to IL-2.

Materials and Methods

Target cells Yac (H-2^a), a murine lymphoma cell line, was propagated in RPMI-1640 culture medium supplemented with 10% fetal calf serum (FCS), 2×10^{-5} M 2-mercaptoethanol, 300 μg/ml glutamine and 60 μg/ml gentamicin (complete medium).

Effector cells Spleen from C57Bl/6 mice were cultured at 5×10^6 with different doses of IL-2 (0–200 U/ml). After two days the cultures were split into two and supplemented with equal volume of fresh medium and IL-2. Activated cells were harvested after five days. Paraformaldehyde fixed tumor cells were obtained by suspending the cells in 1% paraformaldehyde for 5 minutes on ice. Fixed cells were washed three times, counted and added to effector cell cultures during the activation phase.

Cytotoxicity assay Chromium release assay of cytotoxicity was performed as before [9]. Briefly, target cells were labelled with Cr^{51} by incubating 1-2 $\times 10^6$ with 0.1 mCi of sodium chromate solution in normal saline (sp. activity 0.1 Ci/mg chromium, from Bhabha Atomic Research Center, Trombay) and 50 μl of fetal calf serum for 1 hr at 37 °C. Labelled cells were washed three times and suspended in RPMI-1640 with 2% FCS at a density of 1×10^5 cells/ml. Variable number of effector cells along with 10^4 (Cr^{51})-labelled target cells were placed in a well of a 96-well round bottom microtiter plate. Total incubation medium (RPMI-1640 with 2% FCS) in each plate was 0.2 ml. The assay plates were then centrifuged at 500 rpm for 5 min and incubated at 37 °C in a humidified atmosphere of 5% CO_2 and 95% air for 4 hours. After incubation, 0.1 ml of supernatant was removed from each well without disturbing the cells, and the radioactivity level was determined in a LKB gamma counter. Spontaneous release (SR) was determined by incubating target cells in the absence of effector cells. Maximum release (MR) was determined by incubating target cells with 20 μl of 1% Triton X-100 and 80 μl of water. Percent target lysis was calculated using the formula:

$$\% \text{ Target lysis} = (ER-SR)/(MR-SR) \times 100$$

Results

IL-2 activation of mouse spleen NK cells Activation of mouse spleen NK cells in response to IL-2 is a well known phenomenon. Our previous results have indicated that IL-2 induced NK activation in mouse spleen cells is optimal on day 5 [10, 11]. In order to standardize the dose of IL-2 mouse spleen cells were cultured with different doses of IL-2 for 5 days, with a change in medium of day 2, and cytotoxic activity generated against the NK cell target YAC, was examined at several effector: target ratios. Results in Fig. 1 indicate that 20 U/ml of IL-2 (lowest IL-2 dose tested) significantly boosted anti YAC NK activity. Higher doses of IL-2 were more effective and the maximum effect was observed at a dose of 200 U/ml of IL-2.

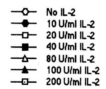

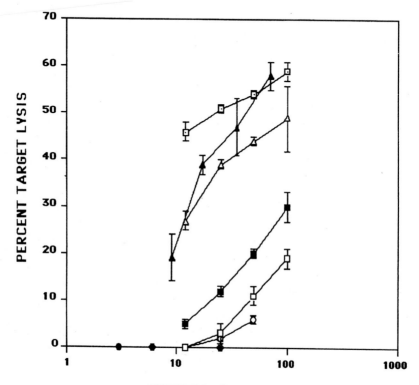

Fig. 1.   Dose response of the effect of different doses of IL-2 on anti-YAC NK activity of mouse spleen cells. Mouse spleen cells were cultured with different doses of IL-1 (0-200 U/ml) for 5 days, as described in methods. The cytotoxic activity of the cultured effector cells against YAC target cells was determined at several E/T ratios. Each value is mean ±SD of three replicate observations.

Effect of fixed tumor cells on NK activity   In order to investigate the effect of tumor target cells on NK cell activity, we attempted to culture mouse spleen cells with tumor target cells. These experiments were unsuccessful as tumor cells rapidly grew in these cultures. When tumor cells were irradiated (1000 rads, gamma irradiation) to prevent the proliferation of tumor cells, we found that such tumor cells were toxic to spleen cells in culture. In order to circumvent this problem, paraformaldehyde fixed tumor cells were used in coculture experiments. Results in Table 1 indicate that coculture of paraformaldehyde fixed tumor cells with mouse spleen cells did not result in any activation of spleen NK cells.

Table 1. Effect of culturing with fixed tumor cells on the NK activity in mouse spleen cells

Effector/Target ratio	Percent target lysis ($\pm$ SD)	
	Spleen cells cultured alone	Spleen cells cultured with fixed tumor
50 : 1	13 ± 3	15 ± 3
25 : 1	9 ± 2	11 ± 2
12 : 1	4 ± 3	7 ± 2
6 : 1	3 ± 1	4 ± 2

Mouse spleen cells were cultured alone or in the presence of fixed tumor cells for 5 days. The cytotoxic activity against YAC target cells was determined by the chromium release assay.

NK cell activation by IL-2 and fixed tumor cells Even though fixed tumor cells did not activate NK cells we tested the effect of fixed tumor cells on NK activation in response to IL-2. In these experiments mouse spleen cells were cultured with 50 and 200 U/ml of IL-2, in the presence or absence of paraformaldehyde fixed tumor cells (tumor to spleen ratio 1: 100). Results in Fig. 2 (A) and (B) clearly indicate that fixed tumor cells boosted remarkably NK cell activation in response to IL-2 at both doses of the cytokine.

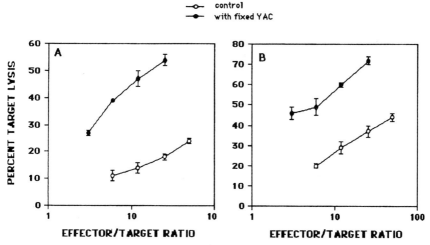

Fig. 2. Anti-YAC cytolytic activity in spleen cells activated with IL-2 in the presence of fixed YAC tumor cells. Mouse spleen cells were activated in vitro with IL-250 U/ml (panel-A) and 200 U/ml (panel-B) for 5 days, either alone (○) or in the presence (●) of paraformaldehyde fixed YAC tumor cells. The tumor to spleen ratio during activation was 1:100. The cytotoxic activity against YAC target cells was determined by the chromium release assay. Each value is mean ± SD of three replicate observations.

Discussion

T cells express IL-2 receptors after sensitization with specific antigens. These high affinity IL-2 receptors comprise three chains (α, β and γ), two of which (β and γ) are members of the cytokine receptor family [4]. NK cells on the other hand constitutively express low affinity receptors for IL-2, which lack the α chain. Differences in the constitution and expression of IL-2 receptors on T cells and the NK cells explain why T cells only respond to IL-2 after sensitization with antigens and respond to very low doses of IL-2. NK cells which do not belong to adaptive immune system and therefore do not require sensitization with a particular antigen for expressing their cytolytic activity, nonetheless respond to high doses of IL-2. T cells recognize antigens by specific T cell receptors which recognize antigenic peptides associated with MHC class I molecules on target cells. Receptors on NK cells which participate in target recognition have not been charcterized but on the basis of competition experiments, it appears that NK cells may also have some sort of target preference [11–14]. What ever be the target recognition receptor on NK cells, the question posed in the present study was, whether singalling through this receptor can activate NK cells? Here by activation, we do not mean the triggering of NK cells, but refer to the induction of higher cytolytic activity, as happens in response to IL-2. Our results indicate that co-culture of NK cells with paraformaldehyde fixed tumor target cells (YAC tumor cells) did not enhance the levels of anti-YAC cytolytic activity. Interestingly howerver, NK activation in response to IL-2 was markedly boosted by simultaneous exposoure to pareformaldehyde fixed tumor target cells. It is well known that sensitized T cells can be induced to proliferate in presence of IL-2 and antigens. If we consider tumor cells as antigens, our results in the present study indicate that NK cells can also get activated by antigens as is the case with T cells. This observation raises several questions. Is NK activation in response to IL-2 and tumor cells due to proliferation of NK cells or their activation or both? Secondly, as NK cells also have some target preference, is NK activation in response to tumor cells and IL-2 specific to the tumor cell used for activation? Finally, what is the mechanism of tumor cell induced boosting of NK activation? Mechanism of signal transduction through IL-2 receptors is different from that of signal transduction through some putative target recognition receptors on NK cells [8]. It will be very interesting to determine if the two signal transduction mechanisms can synergize in NK cells. These experiments are underway in our laboratory.

Acknowledgment

This study was supported by DBT and CSIR grants to RKS. SD received UGC fellowship.

References

1. Lotze, M.T., Grimm, E.A., Mazumdar, A., Strausser, J.L. and Rosenberg, S.A. 1981. Lysis of fresh and cultured autologous tumor by human lymphocytes cultured in T-cell growth factor. *Cancer. Res.* **41:** 4420.
2. Rosenstein, M., Yron, I., Kaufmann, Y. and Rosenberg, S.A. 1984. Lymphokine activated killer cells: Lysis of fresh syngeneic natural killer-resistant murine tumor cells by lumphocytes cultured in interleukin-2. *Cancer. Res.* **44:** 1946.
3. Saxena, R.K., Saxena, Q.B. and Adler, W.H. 1984. Interleukin-2 induced activation of natural killer activity in spleen cells from young and old mice. *Immunology.* **51:** 719.
4. Minami, Y., Kono, T., Miyazaki, T. and Taniguchi, T. 1993. The IL-2 receptor complex: its structure, function and target cells. *Ann. Rev. Immunol.* **11:** 245.
5. Towsend, A., Gotch, F.M. and Davey, J. 1985. Cytotoxic T cells recognize fragments of influenza nucleoprotein. *Cell.* **42:** 457.
6. Yokoyoma, M. and Seaman, W.E. 1993. The Ly-49 and NKR-P1 gene families encoding lectin-like receptors on natural killer cells: the NK gene complex. *Ann. Rev. Immunol.* **11:** 245.
7. Vely, F., Olcese, L., Blery, M. and Vivier, E. 1996. Function of killer cell inhibitory receptors for MHC class I molecules. *Immunol. Letters.* **54:** 145.
8. Biassoni, R., Cantoni, C., Falco, M., Verdiani, S., Bottino, C., Vitale, M., Conte, R., Poggi, A., Moretta, A. and Moretta L. 1996. The Human LeukocyteAntigen (HLA)-C-specific "activatory" or "inhibitory" natural killer cell receptors display highly homologous extracellular domains but differ in their transmembrane and intracytoplasmic portion. *J. Exp. Med.* **183:** 645.
9. Saxena, R.K. and Adler, W.H. 1979. Modulation of natural cytotoxicity by alloantibodies. I. Alloantisera enhancement of cytotoxicity of mouse spleen cells towards a human myeloid cell line *J. Immunol.* **123:** 846.
10. Sarin A. and Saxena, R.K. 1989. Interleukin-2 induced changes in the buoyant density of cytotoxic cells and its relationship with proliferative activily. *Nat. Imm. and Cell Growth Reg.* **8:** 279.
11. Haridas, V. and Saxena, R.K. 1995. Role of major histocompatibility complex class I antigens in modulating the performance of murine tumor cells in cold target competition assays. *Immunology.* **84:** 86.
12. Saxena, R.K. 1996. Understanding inverse correlation between the levels of class I major histocompatibility complex antigens on tumor cells and their susceptibility to Natural Killer cells: Evidence ofcompetition experiments. Current Science, **70:** 143.
13. Saxena, R.K. 1997. Missing self by heterogeneous NK cells *J. Biosciences* **22:** 3.
14. Saxena, R.K. 1997. Ontogeny of inhibitory receptors for MHC molecules on NK cells. *Immunology Today* **18:** 146.

Immunopharmacology: Strategies for immunotherapy
S.N. Upadhyay (Ed)

8. Immunopharmacologic Modulation of Host Response to Increase Therapeutic Index of Drugs

P.K. Ray, Tanya Das, V. Subbulakshmi, A.K. Ghosh, Gaurisankar Sa, Pratima Sinha and Jayati Sengupta
Immunotechnology and Animal Physiology Sections, Bose Institute,
Calcutta 700 054, India

Introduction

In our day to day life we are exposed to myriad of man-made chemical compounds and products developed by man's synthetic ingenuity. Numerous of those chemicals or drugs are toxic to the mammalian system beyond certain concentration. But it is interesting to note that minor toxic insults do not normally jeopardize our physiological system. In fact, each organism has the built-in capacity to tolerate each chemical, but only up to a certain concentration, what is known popularly as "threshold dose". This varies from chemical to chemical, and also depend to a great extent on the individual concerned. Thus, if the host is competent to fight out such toxic hazards, it should be able to keep itself fit in the otherwise hostile environment.

Sometimes due to continuous exposure to toxic chemicals, drugs or their metabolites, or during the diseased condition, body's intrinsic regulatory program fails—leading to physiological catastrophe. One of the outstanding problems of treatment with chemotherapeutic agents is the toxic reactions of the parent compound or its metabolites. On several occasions, it is observed that the patients fall victims to associated secondary toxicological disorders during chemotherapy, and even die due to the toxicity of the drugs than from the disease itself.

This problem remained a bottleneck over the years due to the lack of development of appropriate regimens of chemotherapy which would provide therapeutic benefit without causing toxicity. In fact, many chemicals and drugs were observed to depress both phase I and phase II biotransformation and detoxification enzyme systems, which otherwise are required to transform and detoxify toxic metabolites. Toxic intermediates also inhibit the bioelimination process (the scavenging cells) and thus come in the way of eliminating the unwanted toxic chemicals and their metabolic products from the body. Moreover, the major defence system of our body, i.e. immune system, also gets functionally suppressed as a result of various disease processes in one hand and also due to the direct toxic effects of chemicals/drugs or their metabolites. As a result when all those intrinsic defence capabilities are grossly compromised, the host loses its fitness for survival. Therefore, unless the entire chemical stress resistance system, if which the immune system of the body plays a vital role, could be stimulated, the fatal effects of toxic and/or carcinogenic chemicals cannot be adequately dealt with. It should also be kept in mind that certain amount of tissue or cellular damages are almost always effected by various toxic drugs. The host ability to repair the damage in an accelerated manner and/or regenerate the depleted cells quickly decides the continuity of species survival. Once all the disorders and damages could be reversed, the host should be able to maintain its 'homeostatic' phenomena for its own survival.

Immunopharmacologic Work Done in the Laboratory

Our laboratory, for the last few decades, had been engaged in finding out how to reduce the associated toxicity of various chemicals/drugs so that the therapeutic index of the drug could the increased by elimination/minimizing its toxicological effects. It has also been analyzed whether or not decreasing the toxicological potency of chemicals, its carcinogenic potency could also be lessened.

Intensive research has been conducted on Protein A (PA), a cell wall protein of *Staphylococcus aureus*. This protein has the unique property to bind with the Fc fragments of immunoglobulin G (IgG) and thus has long been used as an immunological reagent in the laboratory for isolation and separation of IgG from the heterogeneous mixtures. We used this Fc-binding property of PA to absorb out blocking immune complexes from the serum of tumor bearing host. The immunosuppressive "blocking factors" inhibit the host immune system to fight out cancer. We have been successful to remove those blocking factors from rat, dog and human [1–9] tumor bearing hosts, using PA-containing, heat killed and formaline stabilized *S. aureus* as immunoadsorbent. This had caused immunopotentiation and tumor regressing effects in tumor bearers. Later, PA itself was found to cause the same effects, i.e. regression of tumors and immunopotentiation [10–14]. This was later confirmed by various other laboratories [15–19] all over the world.

Amelioration of Toxicity by Protein A

It is very often observed that in case of acute ailment or during chronic therapy, high dose of drugs or a low dose administered over a period of time, is required to control the disease processes. In many of these cases, toxicological problems ensue, causing secondary toxic effects to non-target sets, leading to metabolic malfunctions, decreased hematological profile, depressed immune function and therefore increased susceptibility to infections etc. Toxic metabolites may also affect the genome causing various mutagenic, teratogenic and carcinogenic changes. Drugs used for long-term treatment of cancer, immunosuppressive therapy in transplant recipients, long term treatment of AIDS patients and patients with neurological disorders, autoimmune disorders etc. most often experience systemic disorders of kidney, liver, hematological malfunctions, immunological depression, neurological abnormality, cardio-pulmonary dysfunction etc. But, in order to provide immediate relief to a suffering individual, clinicians have no choice but to follow the conventional modalities of treatment. They withdraw the treatment when toxicity becomes manifest. The disease symptoms progressively increase and the patient dies.

During our search for a biological response modifier, which can increase the therapeutic index of drugs by reducing drug-related toxicity, we had a chance observation that a very small amount of PA could reduce the toxicity of cyclophosphamide [20]. An extension of this study in cases of such as carbontetrachloride [21], benzene [22], aflatoxins [23], *Salmonella* endotoxins [24] etc. should consistent decrease of toxicity of all these toxic compounds.

In all these cases, prior incuolation of a very small amount of PA could render the host the ability to withstand larger than normal dosages of those drugs and chemicals. It was further observed that PA stimulated the cytochrome P450-dependent enzymes of the hepatic microsomal mixed function oxygenase system, both at phase I and phase II levels (24–26). Isoforms of glutathione-S-transferases (pi and mu) are significantly activated after PA treatment [22, 27]. It is postulated that such activation of the Cyt P450 dependent enzymes, by PA helps the host to quickly metabolize and detoxify the toxic metabolic intermediates. The activation of the reticuloendothelial system by PA particularly cells of the monocytes and PMN lineages helped in the elimination of the toxic metabolites in an accelerated manner. In this way, PA rendered increased resistence to the host against toxic and/or carcinogenic molecules. Stimulation of the host immune system by PA, particularly the phagocytes and lymphocytes, results in increased elicitation of various cytokines, i.e. IL1, IL2, IFN-γ, TNF-α etc. [28–32], and possibly some growth factors. This help in replenishment of the host immunocytes and also in regeneration of other cell types.

This is now clear that accelerating the process of detoxification and elimination of toxic chemicals, may help the host in reducing the toxicity and carcinogenicity of any chemical. In fact, we have observed that PA is an effective anticancer agent [10–14]. It could cause regression of 7, 12 dimethyl benzanthracene-induced tumor in rats and mice [9, 10]. All these findings tempted us to hypothesize that potentiation of the intrinsic resistance mechanisms of the host would help in increasing the therapeutic index of any drug, by eliminating their toxic effects in a substantial manner.

Effect of Protein A in Ameliorating AZT Toxicity of Bone Marrow Progenitor Cells

To further confirm our hypothesis recently we carried out studies with Azidothymidine (AZT), an anti-AIDS drug, which directly affects bone marrow progenitor cells. PA has been observed to be able to regenerate the depleted CFU-E and CFU-GM cells [28]. To specifically study the regeneration of the progenitor cells affected by AZT, we initiated flowcytometric analysis of bone marrow cells from mice treated with AZT. Our results (Fig. 1) show that AZT specifically knocks out a particular population of stem cells (A: control; B: AZT treated). When the mice were treated with PA and AZT in combination, regeneration of that depleted cell population is observed (C: PA+AZT treated). PA itself increases that particular cell population (D: PA treated). These results indicate that PA can reverse the toxic cellulolytic effect of AZT by replenishing the depleted population of bone marrow progenitor cells. Further

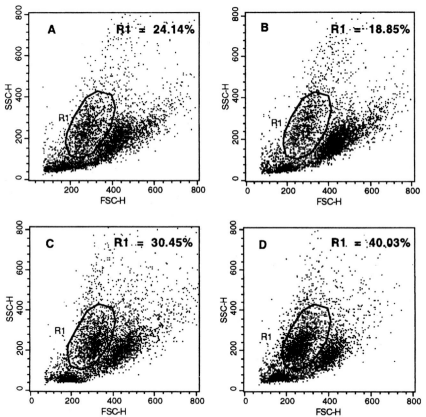

Fig. 1. **Amelioration of AZT-induce toxicity of bone marrow progenitor cells by Protein A. Swiss albino mice were treated with AZT (100 mg/kg) for five days to induce toxicity in the combination group the animals were pretreated twice biweekly with PA (1 μg/20 g body weight) and then with AZT as mentioned above. Control group was exposed to only medium and PA group was inoculated with only PA (1 μg/20 g body weight) twice a week for two weeks. After the last treatment the animals were sacrificed and bone marrow cells were used for flowcytometric analysis. Simultest LeucoGATE was used to reduce debris, if any and dot plot display of ESC (forward scatter due to the size of the cell; x-axis) versus SSC (side scatter due to the granularity of the cell; y-axis) has been shown. A: control; B: AZT; C: PA+AZT; D: PA.**

studies are in progress to identify this cells population as affected by AZT and regenerated by PA.

Erythropoietin: Effects of AZT and Protein A

AZT is already known to cause hematopoietic toxicity [34]. Erythropoietin (Epo) is the hormone essential for the regulation of erythroid progenitor cell production. It was therefore of much importance to study the serum levels of Epo after AZT treatment in presence and absence of Protein A, to understand whether PA can help in reverting AZT-induced anemia or not. Our results showed that serum Epo levels were increased as a result of PA treatment in combination with AZT (Fig. 2). There is a little increase in the AZT group but the change is not significant. It is well known that Epo production increases only during stress conditions. As such, anemic condition due to AZT treatment results in transient increase of Epo production, which is normally observed as a rebound phenomena. But PA group showed much larger increase.

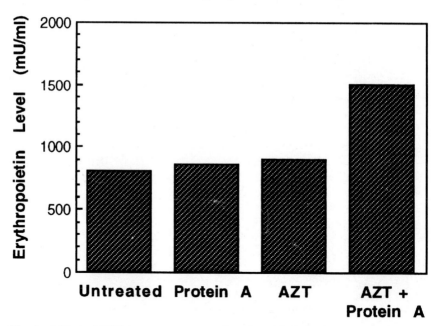

Fig. 2.   Effect of AZT on serum content of erythropoietin in presence or absence of Protein A. Swiss albino mice were treated with AZT (100 mg/kg body weight) for five consecutive days in presence or absence of Protein A (1 μg/20 g body weight biweekly for two weeks). After the last injection blood was collected, serum was separated and analyzed for Epo by ELISA using Epo antibody as raised in the laboratory against standard Protein A.

Effect of Protein A on the Regeneration of the Activity of AZT-inhibited Biotransformation and Detoxification Enzyme System

We have studied the role of PA in ameliorating AZT-related toxic efffects on cytochrome P450 dependent microsomal mixed function mono-oxygenases, including Phase II detoxification enzymes. Our results show that AZT and/ or its metabolites inhibits the activities of cytochrome P450, aminopyrine-N-demethylase, aniline hydroxylase, and also glutathione-S-transferase. In the group of mice treated with PA prior to AZT inoculation, recovery and regeneration of these important enzymes were very much evident (Fig. 3).

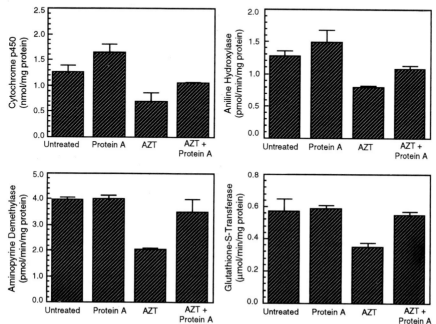

Fig. 3.   Effect of Protein A in ameliorating AZT-induced inhibition of biotransformation enzymes. Swiss albino mice were treated with AZT (100 mg/kg body weight) for five days in the presence of absence of Protein A (1 μg/20 g body weight) biweekly for two weeks. After the last treatment animals were sacrificed, microsomes isolated from liver and (a) Cytochrome P450 content, (b) aniline hydroxylase activity, (c) aminopyrine demethylase activity and (d) glutathione-S-transferase activity were determined. Values are mean $\pm$ SEM (Standard Error Mean) of six individual experiments. The data were analysed using Student's T-test (*$p < 0.001$ compared with control or AZT groups).

Effect of Protein A on the Immune Function

One of the major problems associated with toxicity and/or carcinogenicity of drugs and chemicals is the simultaneous depression of the immune system of the host. Interestingly, PA has been found to have significant immunostimulatory properties [28–33, 35, 36]. PA increases phagocytic response shows [35], increased respiratory burst [36] in macrophages, releasing an increased concentration of IL1 [29]. PA activates ADCC response [9], shows increased NK cell activity [12], and an increased LAK cell activity [30]. It increasingly elicits IL-2, TNF-α and IFN-γ[28–33]. Thus PA potentiates the immunological system of the host in a major way.

Cell Cycle Study by Flowcytometry

In order to understand the mechanism of PA-induced immunopotentiation, we did detailed flowcytometric study. PA has been found to stimulate the proliferation of spleenic lymphocytes as has been observed from the cell cycle data in flowcytometry (Fig. 4). In control spleenic lymphocytes (Upper panel), most of the cells are in G0/G1 phases (87.5%), only 8.6% in S phase and 3.9% in G2/M phases. After PA treatment (Lower panel), G0/G1 phases decreased to 66.2%, whereas S and G2/M phases increase to 21.2% and 12.6% respectively, indicating mild mitrogenic effect of PA in mice spleenic lymphocytes.

Signaling Pathway of Protein A-induced Cell Proliferation

In a study of find out the signaling pathway of PA-induced cell proliferation. We observed that PA transduces its signal from membrane to nucleus via the pathway tyrosine kinasephospholipase γ-inositol triphosphate-Ca^{2+}-protein kinase C etc. to ultimately cause cell proliferation, since inhibitors of tyrosine kinase (genistein), phospholipase C (U73122) and protein kinase C (H7) block cell proliferation effectively (Fig. 5).

Biological Significance of Immunopotentiation by Protein A

After confirming that PA in one hand activates the detoxification enzymes of the host, and on the other stimulates the immune system, we attempted to find out whether or not PA induces the production of different cytokines, since cytokines are known as body's biological response modulators. Increased production of cytokines could be observed in serum of swiss albino mice. Results of Fig. 6 show that PA could induce the production of IL1-α, IL-1β, IL2, TNF-α and IFN-γ in serum. Since all these cytokines are important biological modulators, activation of their production by PA explains some of the multifarious properties of PA.

Molecular Modeling Study on Proteolytic Fragments of Protein A

It can be assumed that PA, being a foreign protein, would be enzymatically (Proteolytically) cleaved *in vivo*. And the small peptide fragments formed may be responsible for various biological properties of PA *in vivo*. Molecular modeling studies have been carried out on this aspects and a 16 amino acid and 20 amino acid residues identified having ability to bind Fc of IgG. Fc binding activity may have some role in inducing various biological properties of PA. Similar approach might help in identifying other active peptide fragments.

Wisconsin sequence analysis package (Genetic Computer Group ver, 8) was used to predict sequences of different peptide fragments produced by tryptic and chymotryptic degradation. Molecular mechanics simulation (DISCOVER program, ver.2.9.7'95) was used to get minimized energy

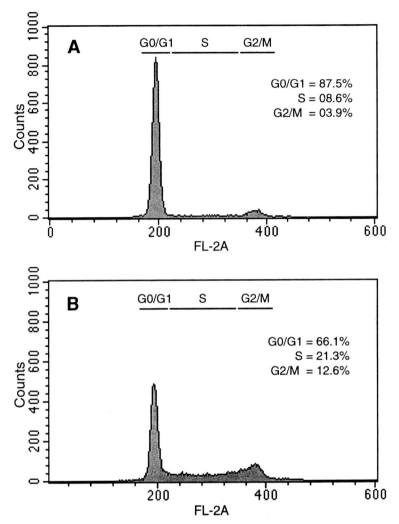

Fig. 4. Cell cycle and DNA content analysis of mice spleenic lymphocytes by flowcytometry. Spleenic lymphocytes of Protein A treated or untreated mice were collected, fixed and nuclear DNA was labeled with PI and cells were analyzed by FACS Calibur. Panels: (A) Spleenic lymphocytes from control mice (B) Spleenic lymphocytes of Protein A treated mice. Simultest LeucoGATE was used to reduce debris, monocytes, granulocytes, if any, and histogram display of FL2-A (x-axis, PI fluorescence) versus counts (y-axis) has been shown.

conformation after orienting these peptides with IgG (Fc) region (docking) properly. Interaction energy (Van der Waals and Electrostatic) for one tryptic fragment (20 amino acid residues) and one chymotryptic fragment (16 amino acid residues) show high binding affinity to IgG (Fc) (Comparable with the interaction taking place for intact B domain of Protein A and IgG for which crystal structure is known [37].

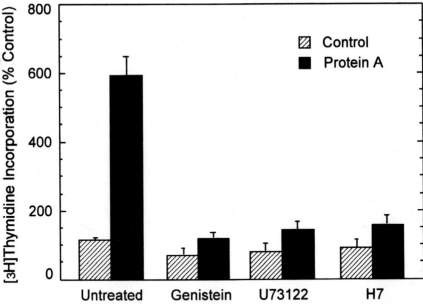

Fig. 5. *Effect of tyrosine kinase, phospholipase C and protein kinase C inhibitors on protein A stimulated spleenic lymphocyte proliferation.* Semiconfluent quiescent spleenic lymphocytes were pretreated with 6 μM genistein, 5 μM U73122 or 2 μM H7 for 90 min at 37°C, then with either medium alone (light striped bars) or with (dark striped bars) 1 μg/ml Protein A. [3H] Thymidine (1 μCi/well) was added during the period 66 to 72 h after initiation of culture. Radioactivity in the TCA-precipitable material was measured as described in Fig. 4. Data are expressed as the mean ± SEM of triplicate cultures.

Discussion

During the last few decades the medical research had experienced many exciting and successful developments. However, in the area of chemotherapy the main limitations prevailed because of (a) susceptibility of the host towards the toxicity of different drugs as well as their metabolites, (b) the improper or less than functional metabolic system in the patient and (c) depressed immune status of the body. As a result, the patient cannot tolerate long-term therapy. The metabolic system gets upset, the immune system falls flat, the intrinsic biological regulation becomes grossly compromised. The host eventually succumbs to death. During the acute phase of any disease or during chronic illness, the clinicians have no other choice but to administer the available required dosages of drug. To find a solution to this unavoidable problem, we thought that, if the biotransformation and detoxifying system of the host could be potentiated, even after its depression due to the toxic drug metabolites, and if the depressed immune system could be activated, the therapeutic index of the drug perhaps would be increased. As a consequence, the drug can be used safely and successfully. Our results in this report are a pointer to this direction and establishes it can be done successfully using a biological response modifier, such as Protein A.

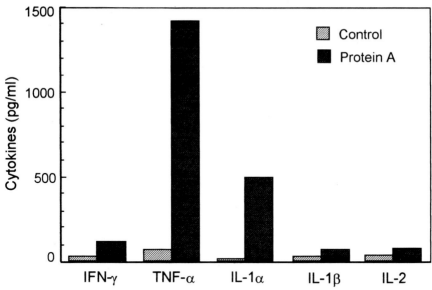

Fig. 6. Production of cytokines by protein A-treated mice spleenic cells. Protein A (10 μg/ml) was injected intravenously to swiss albino mice twice weekly for two weeks. Serum was colected at different time points after last inoculation, in which cytokines were measured by ELISA. Data represents pg/ml individual cytokines over untreated control. Light striped bars represent control system and dark striped bars represent Protein A treated system.

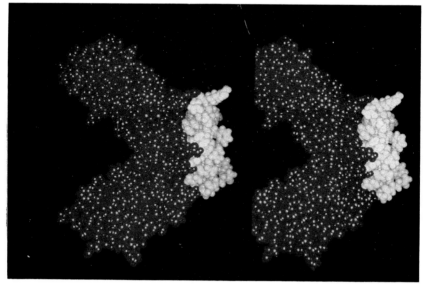

Fig. 7. Stereo drawing of space filling model of IgG and 20 amino acid peptide. Minimized energy conformation of IgG (Fc)* and 20 amino acid peptide* fragment (tryptic digest) complex shows high binding affinity from interaction energy point of view. Immunoprecipitation study confirmed it.

Results of our studies with AZT showed that PA could increase the level of Epo, an important growth hormone for hematopoietic progenitor cells, and thus reversed the loss of hemato-poietic cells due to AZT. The host regained the lost ability to abrogate the toxic effects of AZT. Moreover, by stimulating the production of cytokines, PA could improve the overall intrinsic defence system of the host. These findings help in our understanding that such type of biological response modifier, in combination with or prior to the toxic drug incorporation, might increase the therapeutic index of the drug, by decreasing toxicity and simultaneously repairing the toxic damages in an effective manner.

Molecular modeling study shows that tryptic and chymotryptic digested peptide fragments retain IgG binding property. A 16 amino acid (chymotryptic fragment) and 20 amino acid (tryptic fragment) residues of PA (theoretically predicted) have been already established by us as retaining IgG binding capacity by immunoprecipitation along with capillary electrophoresis analysis.

Conclusion

This observation assumes great importance from the point of view of the fact that drug therapy almost always has its side effects. Reducing the associated toxicity of any drug, of course without diminishing its medicinal potency, drug therapy can be made more useful. Such an approach would revolutionise the second generation chemotherapy to benefit the hypothesis would be of much help to mankind. Our design such formulations, and/or the strategy of future chemotherapy regimens.

Theoretical prediction shows, proteolytically degraded fragments may act as a substitute of whole Protein A molecule with respect to IgG binding property as well as other biological activities (shown by PA). Experimental studies in support to this is needed, which is in progress.

Acknowledgement

The authors acknowledge Mr. U. Ghosh for technical assistance and Mrs. R. Das for typing the manuscript.

References

1. Ray, P.K., Besa, E., Idiculla, A. and Rhoads, J.E. Jr. 1980. *Cancer* **45:** 2633.
2. Ray, P.K., Beas, E., Idiculla, A., Rhoads, J.E. Jr., Bassett, J.G. and Cooper, D.R. 1980. *Clin. Exp. Immunol.* **42:** 308.
3. Ray, P.K., McLaughlin, D., Mohammed, J., Idiculla A., Rhoads, J.E. Jr., Mark, R., Bassett, J.G. and Cooper, D.R. 1981. In "Immune complexes and plasma exchanges in cancer patients" edited by B. Serrou and C. Rosenfeld, Elsevier/North-Holland Biomedical Press. **1:** 197.
4. Ray, P.K., Idiculla A., Mark, R., Rhoads, J.E. Jr., Thomas, H., Bassett, J.G. and Cooper, D.R. 1982. *Cancer* **49:** 1800.

5. Ray, P.K., Raychaudhury, S. and Allen, P. 1982. *Cancer Res.* **42:** 4970.
6. Ray, P.K. and Bandhyopadhyay, S. 1983. *Immunol. Cummun.* **12:** 453.
7. Ray, P.K., Mohammed, J., Allen, P., Raychaudhury, S., Dohadwala, M., Bandhyopadhyay, S. and Mark, R. 1984. *J. Biol. Resp. Modif.* **3:** 39.
8. Ray, P.K. 1985. In: Contemporary topics in immunobiology (F.A. Salinas and M.G. Hanna, Jr., Eds.), Plenum Publishing Corp., N.Y. **15:** 147.
9. Ray, P.K. and Bandhyopadhyay, S. 1985. *Cancer* **56:** 266.
10. Kumar, S., Shukla, Y., Prasad, A.K., Verma, A.S., Dwivedi, P.D., Mehrotra, N.K. and Ray, P.K. 1992. *Cancer Lett.* **61:** 105.
11. Ray, P.K., and Srivastava, M. 1996. *Cancer J.* **9:** 221.
12. Dwivedi, P.D., Verma, A.S. and Ray, P.K. 1992. Immunopharmacol. *Immunotoxicol.* **14:** 105.
13. Ray, P.K., Bandyopadhyay S., Dohadwala, M., et al. 1984. *Cancer Immunol. Immunother.* **18:** 29.
14. Shukla, Y., Verma, A.S., Mehrotra, N.K. and Ray, P.K. 1996. *Cancer Lett.* **103:** 41.
15. Bansal, M.R., Khanna, D., Gupta, K.G. and Jain, P.K. 1989. *Environ. Pathol. Toxicol. Oncol.* **9:** 343.
16. Bansal, M.R., Jain, P., Gupta, K.G. and Khanna, D. 1992. *Environ. Pathol. Toxicol. Oncol.* **11:** 43.
17. Bensinger, W.I., Kinet, J.B., Hennen, G., Franckenne, F., Schaus, C., Saint-Remy, M., Hoyous, P. and Mathieu, P., 1982. New Engl. *J. Med.* **306:** 935.
18. Harper, H.D., Sjoquist, J., Hardy, W.D. Jr. and Jones, F.R. 1985. *Cancer* **55:** 1863.
19. Messerchmidt, G.L., Bowles, C.A., Henry, D.H. and Deisseroth, A.B. 1984. *J. Biol. Resp. Modif.* **3:** 325.
20. Ray, P.K., Dohadwala, M., Bandyopadhyay S., Canchanapan, P. and McLaughlin, D. 1985. *Cancer Chemo. Pharmacol.* **4:** 59.
21. Singh, K.P., Zaidi, S.A., Raisuddin, S., Sazena, A.K., Dwivedi, P.D., Seth, P.K. and Ray, P.K. 1990. *Toxicol. Lett.* **51:** 339.
22. Shankar, U., Kumar, A. Rao, G.S., Dwivedi, P.D., Pandya, K.P. and Ray P.K. 1993. *Biochem. Pharmacol.* **46:** 517.
23. Raisuddin, S., Singh, K.P., Zaidi, S.A. and Ray, P.K. 1994. *Int. J. Immunopharmacol.* **16:** 977.
24. Dwivedi, P.D., Verma, A.S., Mishra, A., Singh, K.P., Prasad, A.K., Saxena, A.K., Dutta, K.K., Mathur, N. and Ray, P.K. 1989. *Toxicol. Lett.* **49:** 1.
25. Dohadwala, M. and Ray, P.K. 1985. *Cancer Chemo. Pharmacol.* **4:** 2002.
26. Srivastava, S.P., Singh, K.P., Saxena, A.K., Seth, P.K. and Ray, P.K. 1987. *Biochem. Pharmacol.* **36:** 4055.
27. Dwivedi, P.D., Kumar, A., Prasad, A.K., Pandya, K.P. and Ray, P.K. 1990. *Biochem. Biophys. Res. Commun.* 169: 476.
28. Ray, P.K., Datta, P.K., Das, T., Srivastava, M. and Subbulakhmi, S. 1997. In: Immunomodulation (S.N. Upadhyay, Ed.), Narosa Publishing House, New Delhi, 101.
29. Prasad, A.K. and Ray, P.K. 1991. *Int. J. Toxicol. Environ. Health.* **1:** 101.
30. Singh, K.P., Shau, M., Gupta, A.K., Kopald, K. and Ray, P.K. 1992. *Immunopharmacol. Immunotoxicol.* **14:** 79.
31. Paul, B.N., Saxena, A.K., Ray, P.K. 1993. *Immunol. Infect. Dis.* **3:** 295.
32. Catalona, W.J., Ratcleff, T.L. and McCool, R.E. 1981. *Nature* **291:** 77.
33. Ray, P.K., Goenka, S., Das, T., Sa, G., Sinha, P. and Srivastava M. (In Press) In: Biological oxidants and antioxidants: Molecular mechanisms and health effects (T. Gitler, Ed.), AOCS Press, USA.

34. Richman, D.D., Fischl, M.A., Grieco, M.H., Gottlieb, M.S., Volberding, P.A. Laskin, O.L., Leedom, J.M., Groopman, J.E., Midvan, D. and Hirsch, M.S. 1987 *N. Eng. J. Med.* **317:** 192.

35. Prasad, A.K., Singh, K.P., Saxena, A.K., Mathur, N.K. and Ray, P.K. 1987. *Immunopharmacol. Immunotoxicol.* **9:** 541.

36. Misra, A. Dwivedi, P.D., Verma, A.S. and Ray, P.K. 1992. *Immunology Lett.* **34:** 289.

37. Deisenhofer, J. 1981. *Biochemistry* **20(9):** 2361.

Immunopharmacology: Strategies for immunotherapy
S.N. Upadhyay (Ed)

9. Peptides as Immunomodulators

V.K. Singh, K. Bajpai, S. Biswas, V.C. Dhawan*, A. Rastogi*, R. Sharan*, W. Haq*, K.B. Mathur* and S.S. Agarwal

Sanjay Gandhi Post-Graduate Institute of Medical Sciences, Lucknow-226 014, India

*Central Drug Research Institute, Lucknow-226 001, India

Abstract

Immunemodulators can be broadly defined as substances which have the ability to influence various components of the immune system. They can be used therapeutically for correcting the pathological aberrations of the immune response, or for augmentation/inhibition of physiological responses. The action of the immunomodulators may be on the specific or non-specific components of the immune responses. Endeavours to develop chemically well defined compounds possessing immunomodulating properties have resulted in the identification of several classes of compounds which can act as immuno-stimulators or immunosuppressors.

As part of our ongoing programme on development of small synthetic peptides as potent and non-toxic immunomodulators for clinical use, we undertook the synthesis and evaluation of few analogs of naturally occurring peptides with known immunomodulating activities. We have identified analogs of interleukin-1β (IL-1β) nonapeptide (163–171), met-enkephalin and thymopentin. Amongst those tested, we have found 2IL-1β analogs which have stimulated mouse thymocyte proliferation and inhibited A375 cells *in vitro*. Two analogs of thymopentin were found to augment the human natural killer (NK) cell activity, CD2R expression, IL-2 production, increase antibody response to SRBC and HLA-B7 gene expression. In the case of met-enkephalin too, two analogs have been found to augment human NK cells, T-cell proliferation, IL-2 production and CD2R expression. The activity of met-enkephalin analogs was completely inhibited by naloxone, an opioid antagonist. These studies provide interesting leads for designing novel peptides that may be more suitable for pharmaceutical application in terms of stability, biodisposition, and receptor affinity.

Introduction

Immunemodulators are substances that act on the immune system and have the ability to modify the immune response. Their effects may be stimulatory or suppressive on the basis of which they may be referred to as immunestimulants or immunesuppressants. Immunestimulants that are generally administered along with antigens or vaccines are known as immunoadjuvants. Non-specific immunestimulation is aimed to enhance state of resistance to pathogens or tumors. In this capacity, their use has been proposed along with chemotherapy to combat intracellular/chronic infections, and to eliminate the residual tumor, such as in melanoma, colon cancer and bladder cancer etc. The potential role of immunestimulants to protect against infections, or immune surveillance against cancer, or enhancement of immune deficiency states (primary or secondary, such as AIDS) has not yet been realised. Non-specific immune-suppressants reduce the capacity of the immune system to respond to antigens, either by killing the dividing cells as in the case of cytotoxic drugs and steroids, or by interfering with the processes of signal transduction etc, in a more selective way, as done by cyclosporin A, and rapamycin. These immune-suppressive drugs that selectively block the function of T-lymphocytes have been widely used to prevent graft rejection (also graft vs host disease) and to conrol autoimmune diseases. Theoretically, prophylactic use of safe suppressants could reduce the occurrence of autoimmune disease/allergy in susceptible individuals.

Considering the immense potential of immunemodulators in prevention and control of a variety of disease states, we have been interested in developing small synthetic peptides as potent and non-toxic immunemodulators [1–7]. Some of our recent findings in this area are summarized in this paper.

Interleukin-1β Nonapeptide

Interleukin-1 (IL-1) refers to a family of closely related proteins which are involved in the development and maintenance of inflammatory responses, as well as amplification of both cellular and humoral immune responses to infectious and foreign agents [8]. IL-1 appear to be identical to the endogenous pyrogen which is considered to be responsible for the increase in basal temperature after infectious events which eventually lead to a protective immune response against infection [9, 10]. Furthermore, IL-1 is capable of inducing receptors for IL-2 and colony stimulating factors, which are not only involved in leukocyte growth and differentiation but also in the synthesis and release of IL-2, IL-4, IL-6 and IL-8. It is through this cascade of events that the host immune and inflammatory responses are sustained. IL-1 is also involved and possibly responsible for the development of chronic immunoinflammatory conditions such as rheumatoid arthritis. It also appears to be the mediator of chronic inflammation in degenerative arthropathies [11]. It has been reported to participate in antigen induced T-cell activation and clonal expansion by triggering IL-2 and IL-4 production, and IL-2 receptor expression [12, 13]. IL-1 is one of the factors involved in B cell differentiation and proliferation, and it has hematopoietic activity for the earliest precursors in the bone marrow [14, 15]. It has been suggested that IL-1 may serve as an effective adjuvant in conjunction with weakly immunogenic vaccines but due to numerous side effects associated with the proinflammatory action of IL-1, its clinical application has been restricted.

The structure-function relationship in human IL-1β has been investigated by means of computer prediction, synthesis of its short peptide fragments and use of monoclonal antibodies of pre-determined specificity. Several attempts have been also made to identify the minimal structural unit(s) of IL-1β responsible for eliciting specific biological response(s), in order to get a therapeutically useful peptide [16]. Antoni et al., (1986) synthesized several small peptide fragments of human and murine IL-1β on the basis of their predicted exposure on the surface of the molecules [17]. They found that the nonapeptide Val-Gln-Gly-Glu-Glu-Ser-Asn-Asp-Lys corresponding to the highly hydrophilic fragment 163–171 of human IL-1β had the ability to mimic some of the immunostimulatory activities of IL-1β itself, while it was non-pyrogenic and non-inflammatory. The nonapeptide was also shown to increase the primary and secondary immune responses against T helper-dependent antigen (SRBC) as well as T helper-independent polysaccharide antigen (SIII derived from *Streptococcus pneumoniae*) in mice [18, 19]. Adjuvant activity of this nonapeptide was observed in mice immunodeficient for genetic (nude mice), natural (aged mice) or iatrogenic (radiation or cyclophosphamide treated) reasons [20–22]. IL-β fragment (163–171) was also shown to have adjuvant activity in tumor therapy [23]. It has been suggested that the adjuvant effect *in vivo* is exerted by the intact peptide, rather than by its metabolites [24]. All these observations lead one to believe that discrete domains within the IL-1β polypeptide might be responsible for the different biological activities of the molecule and that the 163–171 fragment may represent one of the sites responsible for the immunostimulating activity of IL-1β [25]. Recently, Siddiqui et al., (1994) emphasised the importance of the conformational features (β-turn and random coil) of the peptide for T-cell stimulation [26].

The activity profile of IL-1β nonapeptide discussed above prompted us to undertake the synthesis and evaluation of some of its novel lipophilic and more stable analogs. Two lipophilic derivatives of this nonapeptide, one having a lauroyl residue ($C_{11}H_{23}CO$-Val-Gln-Gly-Glu-Glu-Ser-Asn-Asp-Lys; 1) and the other having a palmitoyl residue ($C_{15}H_{31}CO$-Val-Glin-Gly-Glu-Ser-Asn-Asp-Lys; 2) at the N-terminus of the peptide, and a more stable analog carrying D-Val residue at position 1 of the peptide (D-Val-Gln-Gly-Glu-Glu-Ser-Asn-Asp-Lys; 3) were initially synthesized with a view to find out if these structural modifications had a favourable effect on *in vitro* mouse thymocyte proliferation and IL-1 dependent inhibition of human malignant melanoma cells A375. We have found that analogs (1) and (2) are active in both the tests like the parent nonapeptide [3]. The lipophilic analog (2) is in fact, effective at a lower dose as compared to the parent nonapeptide in mouse thymocyte proliferation assay. Although the analog (3) has the ability to inhibit A375 cells, it does not stimulate mouse thymocyte proliferation *in vitro* suggesting that different structures may be responsible for stimulation of mouse thymocyte proliferation and inhibition of A375 cells. IL-1β fragment [163–171] and the analog (2) were also compared for their effects on pyrogenicity, blood glucose level, acute phase response and radioprotection [3]. Unlike IL-1β, its fragment [163–171] and the analog (2) do not induce pyrogenicity and any of the acute phase related changes such as the increase in C-reactive protein and hypoglycemia following their administration in BALB/c mice. We have also found that 40% of animals treated with analog (2) survived more than 21 days after lethal irradiation as compared to 20% survivors in groups treated with recombinant IL-1β or its nonapeptide fragment, under conditions when all the control animals died within 10 days [3].

Met-Enkephalin Analogs

The opioid pentapeptides called enkephalins were originally described as the endogenous ligands for the opioid receptors [27]. Although their precise physiological significance still remains elusive, the enkephalins have been reported to exhibit analgesic, antidepressant, antianxiety and anticonvulsant activities [28]. In addition, enkephalins have also been found to act as immunomodulators [29–34]. Met-enkephalin (Tyr-Gly-Gly-Phe-Met) has been shown to prolong the survival time of mice inoculated with L1210 leukemia or B16-BL6 melanoma cells [35] and modulate phagocytosis in mice [36]. Kita et al. (1992) have demonstrated that treatment of mice splenocytes with met-enkephalin *in vitro* increased their lytic activity against human ovarian cancer cells significantly [37]. A combination of met-enkephalin and AZT has been shown to significantly improve the survival of retrovirus infected mice [38]. Although the majority of effects of opioid peptides on immune response are stimulatory in nature, they have certain immunesuppressive properties as well [39–43]. Reports indicating both, stimulatory as well as inhibitory effects of met-enkephalin on NK cell cytotoxicity are also available in literature [44, 45]. Huckelbridge et al. (1990) have reported the proliferation of human peripheral blood mononuclear cells (PBMC) induced by this pentapeptide in the absence of antigen or mitogen stimulation [46]. Met-enkephalin is known to increase CD2R, thereby suggesting that normal human T-lymphocytes bear surface receptors for met-enkephalin [47].

In view of the above findings, we decided to examine the immunemodulating properties of a few potent and longer-acting congeners of met-enkephalin synthesized by us [48]. The amino acid sequences are, Tyr-D-Ala-Gly-MePhe-Met-NHC$_3$H$_3$H$_7$-iso (1), Tyr-D-Ala-Gly-MePhe-Gly-NHc$_3$H$_7$-iso (2), Tyr-D-Ala-Gly-MePhe-Gly-NHCH$_2$C$_6$H$_5$ (3) and Tyr-D-Ala-Gly-ΔPhe-D-Leu-NHNHC$_6$H$_5$ (4). Analogs (1) and (2) have been found to be as potent as met-enkephalin in stimulating human T-cell proliferation and augmenting NK cell cytotoxicity *in vitro* [1]. The analog (3) had no effect on both, the human T-cell proliferation and NK cell augmentation *in vitro*. Analog (4) was, however, found to augment human NK cell *in vitro* but failed to stimulate T-cell proliferation. Proliferative response was measured by ^{3}H-thymidine uptake after 5 days of incubation. The kinetics of T-cell proliferative response were similar to those for *in vitro* T-cell response to specific antigens rather than via polyclonal activation. The stimulation of T-cell proliferation was inhibited by naloxone, an opioid antagonist. The three peptides (met-enkephalin, analog (1) and (2) also enhanced active T-cell rosette (CD2R) significantly on *in vitro* treatment [2]. Furthermore, these analogs stimulated IL-2 production by human PBMC *in vitro* which was completely inhibited by naloxone. It is also important to note that we did not observe biphasic action either with met-enkephalin or its analogs. Our data demonstrate the physiological importance of met-enkephalin and its analogs in modulating human lymphocyte activity. The study also supports the earlier suggestions that human T-cells bear receptor for met-enkephalin on their surface. Analysis of the mechanisms involved in immunemodulation by these peptides using various peptide agonists, antagonists and cloned receptors is under progress.

The pharmacological effects of analog (2) have already been well studied. It is a potent analgesic and has been found to be several times more potent than morphine by central and oral routes [49].

Earlier investigations with analog (2) have shown it to be 2–3 fold more potent than met-enkephalin in elaborating *Plasmodium cynomolgi* antigen induced colony-stimulating factors by macrophages [31]. Moreover, this analog was shown to modulate Con A stimulated phagocytosis-promoting activity in a dose dependent manner in the culture of more splenocytes *in vitro* [32]. At 10^{-6} and 10^{-5} M concentrations, phagocytosis-promoting activity was inhibited and at 10^{-9} and 10^{-7} M concentrations the above activity was augmented. Further evaluation of the opioidergic activity of analog (2) in mice showed that in addition to antinociception (warm water tail flick test), it also produced tolerance, cross tolerance to morphine and physical dependence [50]. The time course of antinociceptive effect of the analog was comparable to morphine. The antinociceptive ED_{50} (μmol/kg, i.p.) values for the analog and morphine base were 5.31 and 7.59, respectively. Its antinociceptive effect was blocked by naloxone, β-FNA (μ antagonist) and naloxonazine (μ_1 antagonist) but not by ICI 174, 864 (δ antagonist). Naloxone precipitated withdrawal jumpings were 2.6 times less in analog (2) treated mice than the morphine treated group. The above study not only confirmed that analog (2) is a potent μ agonist antinociceptive with a possible weak dependence liability, but also points to its suitability for clinical exploitation.

Thymopentin

Splenopentin (SP-5, Arg-Lys-Glu-Val-Tyr) and thymopentin (TP-5, Arg-Lys-Asp-Val-Tyr) are synthetic immunemodulating peptides corresponding to the region 32–36 of a splenic product called splenin (SP) and the thymic hormone thymopoietin (TP), respectively [51, 52]. TP was originally isolated as a 5-kDa (49-amino acids) protein from bovine thymus while studying effects of the thymic extracts on neuromuscular transmission and was subsequently found to affect T-cell differentiation and function. A radioimmunoassay for TP revealed a cross-reaction with a product found in spleen and lymph node [53, 54]. This product, named SP, differed from TP only in position 34, aspartic acid for bovine TP and glutamic acid for bovine SP, and it was called TP III as well. The synthetic pentapeptides (TP-5) and (SP-5) were found to, reproduce the biological activities of TP and SP, respectively [7].

Harris et al. [1994] reported the isolation of cDNA clones for three alternatively spliced mRNAs that encode three distinct human thymopoietins [55]. Proteins encoded by these mRNAs were named TPα (kDa), β (51 kDa), and γ (39 kDa) and contained similar N-terminal regions, including sequences nearly identical to that of the originally isolated thymopoietins, but divergent C-terminal regions [56]. It is now evident that these 49 amino acid proteins were created by proteolytic cleavage of a larger protein during isolation and represent the N-terminal sequences of these proteins. The finding of a single thymopoietin gene suggests that its variant forms purified from thymus and reported in earlier publications may be related to post-translational modifications and/or amino acid sequencing errors. This finding, however, does not support earlier suggestions from protein sequencing that SP is a distinct molecule. Rather, it would now seem that errors in interpretation of amino acid sequence data led to these conclusions and that the TP like material purified from spleen was thymopoietin itself. Thus, peptides reported as analogs of SP-5 in our earlier studies have now been called as TP-5 analogs.

We undertook the synthesis and evaluation of TP 5 analogs with a view to study their immunomodulatory activity. A total of 13 analogs were synthesized and were evaluated for human NK cell augmentation and T-cell proliferation *in vitro:* Lys-Lys-Glu-Val-Tyr (1), D-Lys-Lys-Glu-Val-Tyr (2), Arg-D-Lys-Glu-Val-Tyr (3), Arg-Lys-Gly-Val-Tyr (4), Arg-Lys-Gln-Val Tyr (5) Arg-Lys-D-Glu-Val-Tyr (6), Arg-Lys-Asn-Val-Tyr (7), Orn-Lys-Glu-Val-Tyr (8), Arg-Orn-Glu-Val-Tyr (9), Arg-Lys-Glu-Ile-Tyr (10), Arg-Lys-Glu-Leu-Tyr (11), D-Lys-D-Pro-Val-Tyr (12) and D-Lys-Lys-Pro-Val-Tyr (13). The peptide earlier known as SP-5 and now considered as another analogs of TP-5 (Arg-Lys-Glu-Val-Tyr) was used as the control for comparison. Analogs [1] and [2] were found to stimulate *in vitro* human NK cell cytotoxicity (figure 1). These analogs were also shown to stimulate IL-2 production, CD2R expression and antibody response against SRBC in mice [4]. We have also demonstrated that analogs (1), (2) and (3) are able to upregulate the transcription of HLA-B7 gene in K562 cells. These cells normally do not transcribe the HLA class I genes. Electrophoretic mobility shift assays indicate that this transcriptional up regulation of HLA class I genes may be related to the appearance of novel class I promoter binding factors induced in the nuclei of treated cells [5].

% increase in cytotoxicity

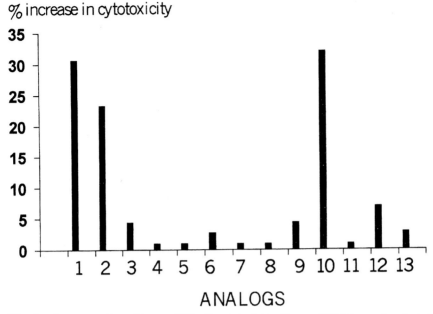

ANALOGS

Fig. 1. Augmentation of human NK cell cytotoxicity. Human PBMC were incubated
with 10^{-4} M concentration of peptides for 18 hr for stimulating effectors.
Cytotoxicity assay was done by ^{51}Cr release assay in triplicate. Assays with
analog (1) and (2) were repeated three times with the PBMC of three different
healthy volunteers and stimulation was found to be consistent and statistically
significant. Analog (10) showed subject (volunteer) related variation.

Conclusion

Significant advances have been made in the study of immunemodulators
during the past two decades. However, the intricacies pertaining to our
knowledge in the field of immunomodulators and their role in the control of
human diseases have just begun to unfold. Additional work will be required
to establish their utility in future. For the present, it would be desirable to
identify suitable immunemodulators which may find use in control, treatment
and prevention of different kinds of diseases. If *in vitro* and *in vivo* results
obtained in various laboratories using different animal models are substantiated,
immunemodulators may provide a new tool for stimulation of innate host
resistance, particularly against cancer, viral and parasitic infections. The studies
reported here constitute an endeavour towards generating new leads for
designing analogs of naturally occurring proteins and peptides so that
compounds more suitable for pharmaceutical applications can be synthesized.

Acknowledgements

The authors thank Mr. Vinod Trivedi for excellent word processing. Financial
assistance from Council of Scientific and Industrial Research, New Delhi is
gratefully acknowledged. The laboratory infrastructure was provided by JICA
grant-in-aid to the SGPGI projects.

References

1. Bajpai K., Singh V.K., Agarwal S.S., Dhawan V.C., Naqvi T., Haq W., Mathur K.B., Immunomodulatory activity of met-enkephalin and its two potent analogs. *Int. J. Immunopharmacol.* 1995; **17**: 207–212.

2. Bajpai, K., Singh V.K., Dhawan V.C., Haq W., Mathur K.B., Agarwal S.S., Immunomodulation by two potent analogs of met-enkephalin. *Immunopharmacology* 1997; **35**: 213–220.

3. Bajpai K., Singh V.K., Sharan R., Haq W., Mathur K.B. Agarwal S.S. Immunomodulatory activity of analogs of interleukin-1β nonapeptides. Immunopharmadcology 1997; **38**: 237–245.

4. Biswas S., Singh V.K., Rastogi A., Haq W., Mathur K.B., Agarwal S.S. Stimulation of IL-2 production and CD2R expression by splenopentin analogs. *Int. J. Immunopharmacol.* 1997; **19**: 341–345.

5. Kishore-Chatterjee M, Agarawal S., Singh V.K., Mathur K.B., Agarwal S.S. Up-regulation of HLA class I gene transcription in K562 cells by analogs of splenopentin (SP-5). *Biochem. Mol. Biol. Intl.* 1997; **41**: 521–528.

6. Rastogi A., Singh V.K., Biswas S., Haq W., Mathur K.B., Agarwal S.S. Augmentation of human natural killer cells by splenopentin analogs. FEBS Lett. 1993; **317**: 93–95.

7. Singh V.K., Biswas S., Mathur K.B., Haq W., Garg S.K., Agarwal S.S. Thymopentin and splenopentin as immunomodulators: Current status. *Immunol. Res.* 1997; **16**: 439–462.

8. Dinarello C.A. The biological properties of interleukin 1. *Eur. Cytokine Net* 1994; **5**: 517–531.

9. Epstein F.H. Interleukin-1 and the pathogens of the acute phase response. *N. Engl. J. Med.* 1984; **311**: 1413–1418.

10. Dinarello C.A. Biological basis for interleukin-1 in disease. *Blood* 1996; **87**: 2095–2147.

11. Pujol J.P., Loyau G. Interleukin-1 and osteoarthritis. *Life Sci.* 1987; **41**: 1187–1198.

12. Lowenthal J.W., Cerottini J.C., MacDonald H.R. Interleukin-1 dependent induction of both interleukin-2 secretion and interleukin-2 receptor expression by thymoma cells. *J. Immunol.* 1986; **137**: 1226–1231.

13. Ho S.N., Abraham R.T., Nilson A., Handwerger B.S., McKeen D.J. Interleukin-1 mediated activation of interleukin-4 producing T. lymphocytes. Proliferation by IL-4- dependent and IL-4-independent mechanisms. *J. Immunol.* 1987; **139**: 1532–1540.

14. Moore M.A.S., Warren D.J. Synergy of interleukin-1 and granulocyte colony stimulating factor: *In vivo* stimulation of stem cells recovery and hematopoietic regeneration following 5-fluorouracil treatment of mice. *Proc. Natl. Acad. Sci. USA* 1987; **84**: 7134–1738.

15. Lipsky P.E. Role of interleukin-1 in human B-cell activation. Contemp. Top Mol. *Immunobiol.* 1985; **10**: 195–217.

16. Mosley B., Dower S.K., Gillis S., Cosman D. Determination of minimum polypeptide lengths of the functionally active sites of human interleukin-1α and 1β. *Proc. Natal. Acad. Sci. USA* 1987; **84**: 4572–4576.

17. Antoni G., Presentini R., Perin F., Tagliabue A., Ghiara P., Censini S., Volpini G., Villa L., oraschi D. A. short synthetic fragment of human interleukin-1 with immunostimulatory but not inflammatory activity. *J Immmunol.* 1986; **137**: 3201–3204.

18. Nencioni L., Villa L., Tagliabue A., Antoni G., Presentini R., Perin F., Silvestrin S., Boraschi D. *In vivo* immunostimulating activity of the 163–171 peptide of human IL-1β. *J. Immunol.* 1987; **139**: 800–804.
19. Lerner U.H., Ljunggren O., Dewhirst F.E., Boraschi D. Comparison of human interleukin-1β and its 163–171 peptide in bone resorption and the immune response. *Cytokine* 1991; **3**: 141–148.
20. Boraschi D., Nencioni L., Villa L., Cesini S., Bossu P., Ghiara P., Presentini R., Perin F., Frasca D., Doria G., Forni G., Musso T., Giovarelli M., Ghezzi P., Bertini R., Besedovsky H.O., Rey A.D., Sipe J.D., Antoni G., Silvestrin S., Tagliabue A., *In vivo* stimulation and restoration of the immune response by the non-inflammatory fragment 163–171 of human interleukin-1β. *J. Exp. Med.* 1988; **168**: 675–686.
21. Frasca D., Boraschi D., Baschieri S., Bossu P., tagliabue A., Adorini L., Doria G. *In vivo* restoration of T-cell functions by human IL-1β or its 163–171 nonapeptide in immunodepressed mice. *J. Immunol.* 1988; **141**: 2651–2655.
22. Tagliabue A., Boraschi D. Cytokines as vaccine adjuvants: Interleukin-1 and its synthetic peptide 163-171. *Vaccine* 1993; **11**: 594–595.
23. McCune C.S., Marquis D.M. Interleukin-1 as an adjuvant for active specific immunotherapy in a murine tumor model. *Cancer Res.* 1990; **50**: 1212–1215.
24. Pessina G.P., Bocci V., Nicoletti C., Becherucci C., Presentini R., Parente L., Villa L., Tagliabue A., Boraschi D. Metabolic behavior and distribution of the synthetic nonapeptide fragment 163–171 of human IL-1β. *Lymphokine Res.* 1990; **9**: 371–379.
25. Boraschi D., Antoni G., Perin F., Villa L., Nencioni L., Nencioni L., Ghiara P., Presentini R., Tagliabue A. Defining the structural requirements of a biologically active domain of human IL-1R β. *Eur. Cytokine. Net.* 1990; **1**: 21–26.
26. Siddiqui Z., Sharma A.K., Kumar S., Kumar A., Bhatt P.N. Conformation of a T-Cell stimulating peptide of interleukin-1β protein: Circular dichroism studies. *Int. J. Biol. Macromol.* 1994; **16**: 259–263.
27. Hughes I., Smith T.W., Kosterlitz H.W., Fothergill L.A., Morgan B.A., Morris H.T. Identification of two related pentapeptides from the brain with potent opiate agonist activity. *Nature* 1975; **258**: 577–579.
28. Plotnikoff N.P., Kastin A.J., Coy D.H., Christensen C.W., Schally A.V., Spirtes M.A. Neuropharmacological actions of enkephalin after systemic administration. *Life Sci.* 1976; **19**: 1283–1288.
29. Plotnikoff N.P., Murgo A.J., Miller G.C., Corder C.N., Faith R.E. Enkephalins: immunomodulators. *Fed. Proc.* 1985; **44**: 112–118.
30. Faith R.E., Liang H.J., Murgo A.J., Plotnikoff N.P. Neuroimmunomodulation with enkephalins: Enhancement of natural killer cell activity *in vitro. Clin. Immunol. Immunopathol.* 1984; **31**: 412–418.
31. Singh P.P., Singh S., Dhawan V.C., Haq W., Mathur K.B., Dutta G.P., Srimal R.C., Dhawan B.N. Enkephalins modulation of *Plasmodium cynomolgi* antigens-induced colony stimulating factors elaboration by macrophages. *J. Biol. Regul. Homeost. Agents* 1991; **5**: 142–146.
32. Singh S., Singh P.P., Dhawan V.C., Haq W., Mathur K.B., Dutta G.P., Srimal R.C., Dhawan B.N. Lymphokines production by concanavalin-A stimulated mouse splenocytes: modulation by met-enkephalin and related peptide. *Immunopharmacology* 1994; **27**: 245–251.
33. Wybran J., Schandene, L., Van Vooren J.P., Vandermoten G., Latinne D., Sonet J., De Bruyere M., Taelman H., Plotnikoff N.P. Immunologic properties of methionine-enkephalin, and therapeutic implications in AIDS, ARC and cancer. *Ann. N.Y. Acad. Sci.* 1987; **496**: 108–114.

34. Mazumder S., Nath I., Dhar M.M. Immunomodulation of human T-cell responses with receptor selective enkephalins. *Immunol. Lett.* 1993; **35:** 33–38.
35. Murgo A.J. Inhibition of B16-BL6 melanoma growth in mice by methionine enkephalin. *J. Natl. Cancer. Inst.* 1985; **75:** 341–344.
36. Marotti T., Rabatic S., Gabrilovac J.A. Characterization of the *in vivo* immunomodulation by met-enkephalin in mice. *Int. J. Immunopharmacol.* 1993; **15:** 919–926.
37. Kita T., Kikuchi Y., Oomori K., Nagata I. Effect of opioid peptides on the tumoricidal activity of spleen cells from nude mice with or without tumors. *Cancer Detect. Prev.* 1992; **16:** 211–214.
38. Specter S., Plotnikoff N., Badley W.G., Goodfellow D. Methionine enkephalin combined with AZT therapy reduce murine retrovirus induced disease. *Int. J. Immunopharmacol.* 1994; **16:** 911–917.
39. Johnson H.M., Smith E.M., Tores B.A., Blalock J.E. Regulation of the *in vitro* antibody response by neuroendocrine hormones. *Proc. Natl. Acad. Sci. USA* 1982; **79:** 4171–4174.
40. Heijnen C.J., Bevers C., Kavelaars A., Ballieux R.E. Effect of α-endorphin on the antigen-induced primary antibody response of human blood B cells *in vitro .J. Immunol.* 1986; **136:** 213–216.
41. Carr D.J.J., Serou M. Exogenous and endogenous opioid as biological response modifiers. *Immunopharmacology* 1995; **31:** 59–71.
42. Roda L.G., Bongiorno L., Trani E., Urbani A., Marini M. Positive and negative immunomodulation by opioid peptides. *Int. J. Immunopharmacol.* 1996; **18:** 1–16.
43. Van den Bergh P., Rozing J., Nagelkerken L. Identification of β-endorphin with opposing effects on rat T-cell proliferation. *Immunology* 1993; **79:** 18–23.
44. Ghanta V.K., Rogers C.F., Hsueh C.M., Hiramoto N.S., Soong S.J., Hiramoto R.N. *In vivo* enhancement of NK cell activity with met-enkephalin and glycyl-glutamine: their possible role in the conditioned response. *Int. J. Neurosci.* 1991: **61:** 135–143.
45. Carr D.J.J., Gebhardt B.M., Paul D. Alpha adrenergic and mu-2 opioid receptors are involved in morphine-induced suppression of splenocyte natural killer activity. *J. Pharmacol. Exp. Ther.* 1993; **264:** 1179–1186.
46. Hucklebridge F.H., Hudspith B.N., Lydyard P.M., Brostoff J. Stimulation of human peripheral 1. ymphocytes by methionine-enkephalin and delta selective opioid analgoues. *Immunopharmacology* 1990; **19:** 87–91.
47. Wybran J., Appelboom T., Famaey J.P., Govaerts A. Suggestive evidence for morphine and methionine-enkephalin receptors on normal human blood T lymphocytes. *J. Immunol.* 1979; **123:** 1068–1070.
48. Mathur K.B., Dhotre B.J., Sharma S.D., Raghubir R., Patnaik G.K., Dhawan B.N. Synthesis and biological activity of Met-Enkephalin analogs. NIDA Res Monograph 198; **1488:** 115–117.
49. Raghubir R., Patnaik G.K., Sharma S.D., Mathur K.B., Dhawan B.N. Pharmacological profile of two new analogues of met-enkephalin. In Recent Progress in the Chemistry and Biology of Centrally Acting Peptides ed. by B.N. Dhawan and R.S. Rapaka, pp. 167–174, Central Drug Research Institute, Lucknow, India, 1988.
50. Nath C., Patnaik G.K., Haq W., mathur K.B., Srimal R.C., Dhawan B.N., Porrecca F: Novel Met-enkephalin analogue: A potent systemic mu agonist antinociceptive agent. *Pharmacol. Res.* 1995; **31:** 269–273.
51. Goldstein G., Scheid M.P., Boyse E.A., Schlesinger D.H., Van Wauwe J. A synthetic

pentapeptide with biological activity characteristic of thymic hormone thymopoietin. *Science* 1979; **204:** 1309–1310.

52. Audhya T., Schlesinger D.H., Goldstein G. Complete amino acid sequences of bovine thymopoietin I, II, III: Closely homologous polypeptides. *Biochemistry* 1981; **20:** 6195–6200.

53. Goldstein G. Isolation of bovine thymin: a polypeptide hormone of the thymus. *Nature* 1974; **247:** 11–14.

54. Goldstein G. Radioimmunoassay for thymopoietin. *J. Immunol.* 1976; **117:** 690–692.

55. Harris C.A., Andryuk P.J., Cline S.W., Chan H.K., Natarajan A., Siekierka J.J., Goldstein G. Three distinct human thymopoietins are derived from alternatively spliced mRNAs. *Proc. Natl. Acad. Sci. USA* 1994; **91:** 6283–6287.

56. Harris C.A., Andryuk P.J., Cline S.W., Mathew S., Siekierka J.L., Goldstein G. Structure and Mapping of the human thymopoietin (TMPO) gene and relationship of human TMPO beta to rat lamin-associated polypeptide 2. Genomics 1995; **28:** 198–205.

Immunopharmacology: Strategies for immunotherapy
S.N. Upadhyay (Ed)

10. Futher Studies on Immunomodulation by Natural Products from *Tinospora cordifolia*

K.B. Sainis, Rupal Ramakrishnan, P.F. Sumariwalla, A.T. Sipahimalani, G.J. Chintalwar and A. Benerji

Cell Biology and Bio-organic Divisions, Bhabha Atomic Research Centre,
Modular Laboratories, Trombay, Mumbai 400 085, India

Tinospora cordifolia, belonging to the family *Menispermaceae*, is an important medicinal plant considered to be a Rasayana, Medhya and anti-ageing drug in the Ayurvedic system of medicine [1]. In recent years oral administration of the aqueous stem extracts of this plant has been shown to protect experimental animals against abdominal infections and sepsis [2–4], improve Kupffer cell function and polymorphonuclear cell (PMN)—mediated phagocytosis in rats with chronic liver damage and patients of surgical jaundice respectively [5, 6] and stimulate colony stimulating factor activity in serum [7]. We have, for the first time, demonstrated a direct effect of the dry stem crude aqueous extract (DSCE-Aq) of *Tinospora cordifolia* on mouse lymphocytes. DSCE-Aq was observed to be polyclonally mitogenic only to B lymphocytes [8, 9]. Activity based purification of this mitogenic principle was also achieved. The present studies were carried out to assess the effects of DSCE-Aq and its active principle on humoral and cell mediated immune responses to specific antigens.

Materials and Methods

DSCE-Aq was prepared as described previously [9]. It was further fractionated using polar and apolar solvents and various chromatographic procedures. All the fractions were screened for mitogenic activity against C3H mouse spleen cells in terms of ^{3}H thymidine incorporation as described earlier [9]. Two preparations called partially purified immunomodulator (PPI) and its purifed constituent G1-4A were used in this study.

C3H mice (6 to 8 week-old) of either sex wer used. They were treated with DSCE-Aq (orally, 100 mg/kg, daily for 15 days) or with PPI/G1-4A ((i.p., single injection 2 or 5 days before immunisation, 12.5 to 50 mg/kg).

Immunisation with sheep erythrocytes (SRBC) was carried out by injection of 2×10^8 SRBC i.p. per mouse. Five days later spleen cells were obtained, RBC were lysed by treatment with 0.83% ammonium chloride solution and anti SRBC humoral response was estimated by enumerating the antibody producing cells using a direct hemolytic plaque forming cell assay [10].

In another experiment, mice were immunised with chicken ovalbumin (C-OVA, 100 μg/mouse) emulsified in Freund's complete adjuvant in the hind foot pads. Seven days later their popliteal lymph nodes were dissected out and lymph node cells (LNC) were restimulated with different amounts of C-OVA *in vitro* for 72 hours in RPMI-1640 tissue culture medium containing 10% CPSR-2 (Sigma). The cultures were pulsed with ^{3}H thymidine for 16 hr and proliferation of LNC was estimated as described previously [9].

The effect of administration of G1-4A to mice on T cell response was determined in terms of *in vitro* proliferative response to the polyclonal mitogen concanavalin A (con A), 5 days after injection of G1-4A and to C-OVA in immune LNC 2 days after the injection of PPI. Response to con A was assessed *in vitro* by co-culturing the spleen cells with DSCE-Aq or PPI/G1-4A and con A (5–12.5 μg/ml/10^6 cells) for 3 days.

Stimulation index (S.I.) for the mitogens was calculated as follows:

S.I. = (CPM in mitogen stimulated cells – CPM in untreated cells)/ CPM in unstimulated cells

Levels of two cytokines, IL-4 and IL-10 were estimated in supernatants of mouse spleen cells cultured *in vitro* with DSCE-Aq for different periods of time using the Pharmingen ELISA kit.

Results

Purification of DSCE-Aq led to isolation of the active fractions PPI and G1-4A. The latter was found to be more strongly mitogenic to spleen cells as evident from higher stimulation index ($\cong$ 54, Fig. 1) obtained in its presence than in the presence of PPI.

Oral administration of DSCE-Aq to mice for 15 consecutive days enhanced the humoral immune response to sheep erythrocytes. The number of IgM plaque forming cells in immunised mice pretreated with DSCE-Aq was 4 times that in DSCE-Aq treated unimmunised controls and about 6 times that in untreated immunised controls (Fig. 2). Similar augmentation of anti-SRBC antibody response was obtained by a single injection of PPI 48 hr before immunisation (Fig. 3). This effect was dose dependent (data not shown).

The T cell response to the mitogen con A was significantly suppressed when DSCE-Aq or PPI or G1-4A were added at the beginning of the culture, even at very low concentrations at which the modulator was not mitogenic (Figs. 4 and 5). Though the total ^{3}H thymidine incorporation was increased at higher concentrations of the immunomodulators, the stimulation due to con A itself appeared to have been suppressed if one took into account the increased proliferation induced by DSCE-Aq/PPI (Figs. 4 and 5). Contrary

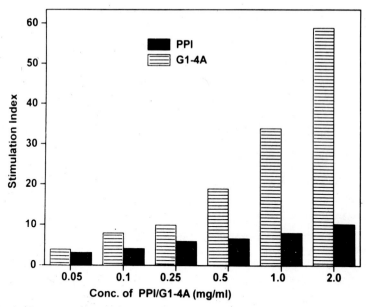

Fig. 1. Response of mouse spleen cells to the mitogenic immunomodulators from *T. cordifolia*.

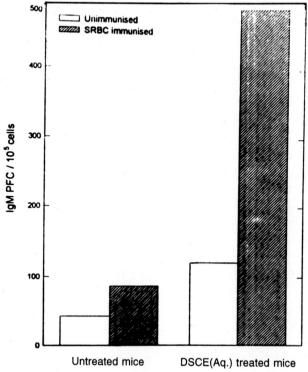

Fig. 2. Effect of oral administration of DSCE-Aq on humoral response to SRBC.

to the *in vitro* effect, treatment of mice with G1-4A *in vivo* enhanced the response of spleen cells to con A *in vitro* (Table 1). This was also evident in the response of the mice to yet another antigen, C-OVA (Fig. 6). A very significantly enhanced proliferative response was seen in C-OVA-immune LNC upon restimulation with the specific antigen.

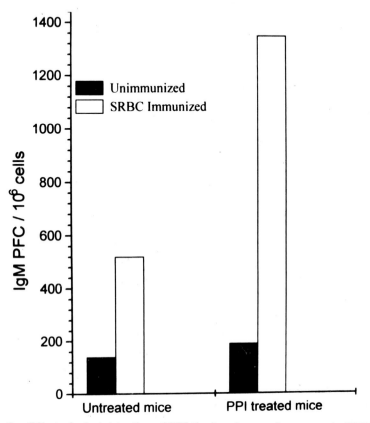

Fig. 3. Effect of administration of PPI (i.p.) on humoral response to SRBC.

The levels of the T_H2 cell cytokines IL-4 and IL-10 estimated in DSCE-Aq stimulated cultures showed reduction when compared with those in unstimulated cells (Figs. 7 and 8).

Discussion

All the earlier reports from other laboratories have demonstrated that the immunomodulatory activity of aqueous stem extracts of *T. cordifolia* was evident mainly in phagocytic functions and both PMN and macrophages appeared to the target cells. Our laboratory, however, identified B lymphocytes as the target cells for the crude extract as well as the purified constituents of *T. cordifolia*. Enrichment of the mitogenic activity was obtained during the purification of G1-4A from the crude DSCE-Aq (Fig. 1). The data presented

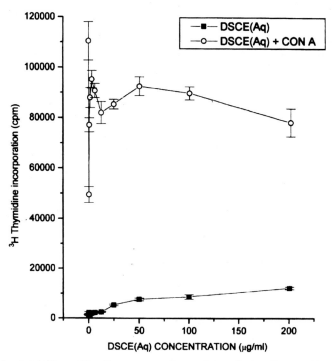

Fig. 4. Inhibition of *in vitro* response to con A in spleen cells co-cultured with DSCE-Aq.

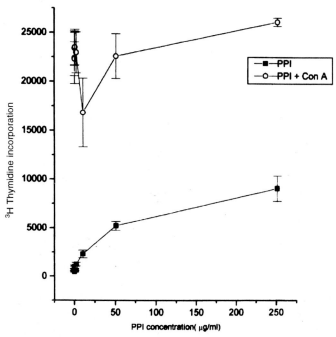

Fig. 5. Inhibition of *in vitro* response to con A in spleen cells co-cultured with PPI.

in the preceding section clearly established that DSCE-Aq and PPI derived from it augmented the humoral response to SRBC (Figs. 2 and 3) when the mice were pretreated with them. A single injection of as low as 12.5 mg. kg PPI was as efficient as 15 day oral administration of DSCE-Aq in this regard.

G1-4A augmented the T cell response to polyclonal mitogen con A when the mice were treated with it *in vivo* (Table 1). The proliferation of C-OVA immune LNC *in vitro* in presence of the specific antigen, which is predominantly a T cell response, was also significantly augmented (Fig. 6). In contrast, these modulators did not enhance but inhibited the T cell response when they were added *in vitro* to the cultures of the spleen cells with con A (Figs. 4 and 5).

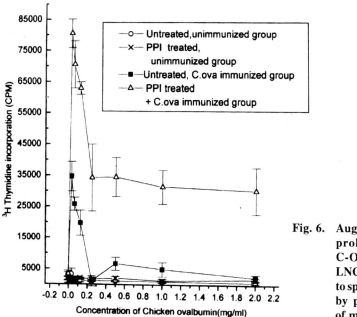

Fig. 6. Augmentation of proliferation in C-OVA immune LNC in response to specific antigen by pre-treatment of mice with PPI.

Thus a clear distinction between the *in vitro* and *in vivo* actions of the *T. cordifolia* derived immunomodulators was visible.

Table 1. Effect of Administration (i.p.) of G1-4A on the Responses of Spleen Cells to Con A *in vitro*

Group	Treatment (i.p.)	^{3}H Thymidine Incorporation Mean CPM ± S.E.M in		
		Cells only	Cells + Con A (5 μg/ml)	Cells + Con A (12.5 μg/ml)
1.	—	1,739 ± 80	86160 ± 7766	11,811 ± 796
2.	G1-4A (12.5 mg/kg)	4,185 ± 457	1,081,56 ± 8559*	19,110 ± 641[a]

Mice were injected G1-4A five days before setting up culture of spleen cells with con A.
^{3}H Thymidine was added to 72 hour cultures
*P < 0.05; a – P < 0.005

It is possible that both macrophages as well as B cells serve as target cells for the action of DSCE-Aq and PPI or G1-4A but the minimum concentration required to activate them may be different. The macrophages are critical for the manifestation of T cell response *in vivo* as well as *in vitro*. The immunomodulatory effects of *T. cordifolia* constituents on T cell responses could ensue from their action on macrophages. They are known to secrete cytokines IL-1 and IL-12 which enhance proliferation of T_H1 cells [11–13]. The B cell too could regulate T_H1 activation through IL-12 [13–14]. Of these cytokines, IL-12 is known to downregulate T_H2 cell functions. The decline in the levels of IL-4 and IL-10 in the supernatants of DSCE-Aq stimulated spleen cells supported such a possibility (Figs. 7 and 8). It may lead only to a switch in the class of IgG synthesised [14]. Consequently, total IgG and IgM levels may remain enhanced while T_H1 cell proliferation which depends on the IL-2 could be augmented provided the stimulating mitogen (con A) is not in some way neutralised. The effect of addition of DSCE-Aq or PPI to the cultures of naive T cells with con A (Figs. 4 and 5) suggest such an interference.

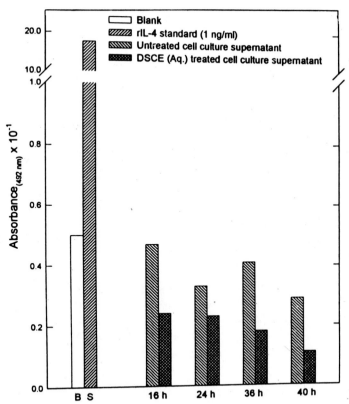

Fig. 7. Level of IL-4 in the supernatants of spleen cells stimulated with DSCE-Aq for different periods of time.

T cells could not be induced to proliferate in presence or absence of macrophages by DSCE-Aq [8, 9]. It may then be argued that the enhancement

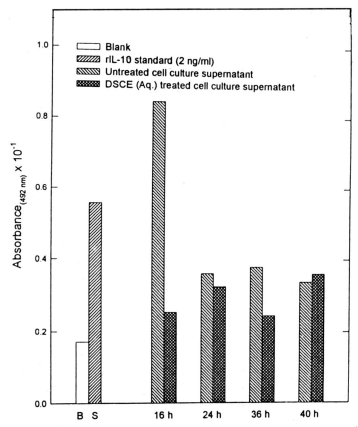

Fig. 8. Level of IL-10 in the supernatants of spleen cells stimulated with DSCE-Aq for different periods of time.

in the proliferative response of immune LNC to C-OVA could be a result of the action of PPI on B cells and not T cells. This will need confirmation using separated T and B cells from the immune LNC. But this argument cannot explain the augmentation of con A induced proliferation in G1-4A treated mice (Table 1), since that is an exclusive T cell phenomenon. Alternatively, one may speculate a role for some non-protein T cell antigens in DSCE. Though DSCE-Aq and PPI contain some amount of protein, G1-4A did not. Thus the opposite immunomodulatory effects of *T. cordifolia* on T cell phenomena *in vivo* and *in vitro* may form an intricate interplay of cytokine interactions.

References

1. Katiyar, C.K., Brindavanan, N.B.,Tiwari, P. and Narayana, D.B. 1997. in "Immunomodulation" ed. S.N. Upadhayay (Narosa Publishing House, New Delhi, India) p. 163.

2. Thatte, U.M., Chhabria, S.S., Karandikar, S.M. and Dahanukar, S.A., 1987. *Indian Drugs*, **75:** 95.
3. Dahanukar, S.A., Thatte, U.M., Pai, N., More, P.B. and Karandikar, S.M. 1988. *Ind. J. Gastroenterol.* **7:** 21.
4. Thatte, U.M. and Dahanukar, S.A. 1989. *Phytotherapy Research.* **3:** 43.
5. Bapat, R.D., Rege, N.N., Koti, R.S., Desai, N.K. and Dahanukar, S.A. 1995. *HPB. Surg.* **9:** 5.
6. Nagarkatti, D.S., Rege, N.N., Desai, N.K. and Dahanukar, S.A. 1994. *J. Postgrad. Med.,* **40:** 65.
7. Thatte, U.M., Rao, S.G.A., and Dahanukar, S.A. 1994. *J. Postgrad. Med.,* **40:** 202.
8. Sumariwalla, P.F., 1996. Ph. D. Thesis, University of Mumbai.
9. Sainis, K.B., Sumariwalla, P.F., Anjali Goel, Chintalwar, G.J., Sipahimalani, A.T. and Benerji, A. 1997. in "Immunomodulation" ed. S.N. Upadhayay (Narosa Publishing House, New Delhi, India.) p. 155.
10. Cunningham, A.J. and Szenberg, A. 1968. *Immunology.* **14:** 599.
11. Rosensterich, D.L., Farrar, J.J. and Dougherty, S. 1976. *J. Immunol.,* **116:** 131.
12. Trinchieri, G. 1993. *Immunology Today.* **14:** 335.
13. Scott, P. 1993. *Science.* **260:** 496.
14. Mosmann, T.R. and Coffman, R.L. 1989. *Ann. Rev. Immunol.* **7:** 145.

Immunopharmacology: Strategies for immunotherapy
S.N. Upadhyay (Ed)

11. Clinical Prospects of *Tinospora cordifolia*: An immunomodulator plant

N.N. Rege, P. Abraham[1], R.D. Bapat[2], V. Ray[3],
U.M. Thatte and S.A. Dahanukar
Departments of Pharmacology and Therapeutics, [1]Gastroenterology, [2]Surgery,
[3]Pathology, Seth G.S. Medical College and KEM Hospital, Mumbai 400 012, India

Introduction

Development of a safe and clinically effective immunostimulant is a major task before today's scientists. Though the voluminous experimental data are available proving immunostimulant properties of many agents, only a few of them have reached the clinic for use in patients. Further, these agents are not freely available, especially in developing countries where they are much needed, are expensive, have to be given parenterally and can lead to serious and disturbing adverse reactions. Hence a vigorous pursuance to develop an immunostimulant continues.

Ayurveda, the traditional system of Indian medicine, is a well developed science of "prevention". It gives a lot of emphasis on the use of therapies that produce a "pro-host" effect, thus keeping a person in a state of "positive health". The plants described as *"rasayana"* in Charaka or Sushruta Samhita are given for prevention of diseases and strengthening of both physical and mental health [1, 2]. They are commonly used following epidemics or during the convalescent period. Using these leads, scientists from India have identified several plants which have been proved to have immunomodulating effects in experimental (*in vitro* systems and *in vivo* models) as well as clinical situations [3].

Tinospora cordifolia, a plant belonging to the *rasayana* group, has been extensively explored in our laboratory for its immunostimulant effects. The stem of this plant has been shown to activate the reticuloendothelial system and polymorphonuclear cells both in *in vitro* and *in vivo* studies [4]. Our findings have been confirmed by other research workers [5, 6]. This plant has also been shown to enhance specific antibody production following immunization with sheep red blood cells and to exhibit concentration dependent polyclonal mitogenic activity [7].

We have developed a standardized, stable formulation from the whole aqueous extract of *Tinospora cordifolia* in collaboration with Merind Ltd.

and have tested it in various clinical disorders associated with the immunosuppression e.g. as an adjuvant to cancer chemotherapeutic agents, in patients with burns, tuberculosis and with liver disorders. This article focuses on the last condition, highlighting the rationale for its selection, the supportive experimental work, the clinical trials conducted and the outcome.

Hepatic Disorders: Need for an immunostimulant

Liver, the custodian of the internal milieu', is continuously exposed to damaging agents, ranging from environmental pollution to an expanding list of hepatotoxic agents—viruses or drugs [8, 9]. Naturally, there is a concern amongst hepatologists to devise ways to protect the liver from various onslaughts. Absence of a breakthrough in developing hepatoprotective agents despite many years of research has resulted in growing interest in folkloric and traditional systems of medicine.

In recent years, rapid progress has been made in understanding the relations existing between various cells of the liver and the pathobiology of cellular events responsible for acute and chronic hepatic damage. An intricate regulatory network has been identified in the liver which maintains the organ in normal state. The chief elements of the network, the parenchymal and non-parenchymal cells (viz. Kupffer cells and Ito cells) of the liver, transduct the signals by depositing extracellular matrix or releasing modulators/effectors [10]. Any disturbance in this signal transduction results in abnormal hepatic reactions manifested as acute or chronic liver damage [11].

Of the three key cells of the liver, the Kupffer cells are the most versatile. These cells are closely linked with host defences. The activity of these cells is a major determinant of outcome of any liver injury. It has been reported that excess activation of Kupffer cells damages the liver [12–14] while hepatic fibrosis is linked with suppressed or subnormal activity of these cells [15]. Thus, modulation of Kupffer cell activity would be a new weapon against liver disorders. However, this therapeutic option has not been explored in depth.

Hepatotherapeutic Potential of *Tinospora cordifolia*

Ancient textbooks of Ayurveda advocate *Tinospora cordifolia* to treat jaundice, to reduce liver and spleen enlargement, and to facilitate bile flow in the presence of obstructive lesions [16–18]. This plant is an ingredient of more than one-third of hepatoprotective formulations available in the Indian market [19]. It is also prescribed as a single entity [20].

To validate the claims of its hepatoprotective effects, we planned laboratory studies using *in vivo* animal models of acute and chronic liver damage (simulating viral hepatitis, fatty infiltration and cirrhosis). Treatment with *Tinospora cordifolia* given prior to administration of hepatotoxins like carbon tetrachloride or galactosamine resulted in aggravation of the liver damage. However, if given concurrently or following the hepatotoxin, it effectively prevented deposition of fibrous tissue and preserved the parenchymal tissue [21–23].

This differential activity of the plant [21, 22] and the immunostimulant potential [4] led us to conduct further studies to find out whether *Tinospora cordifolia* can modify the prognosis of liver diseases associated with immunosuppression.

For this a series of experiments was carried out in a sequential manner. In the beginning, activation of the mononuclear phagocyte system was identified as a key mechanism for the immunostimulant effect of the drug, then a link between the activity of the mononuclear phagocyte system and abonormal hepatic reaction was established. Lastly, *in vivo* model systems were used to verify the effects of the drug on Kupffer cells. These experiments are descibed in short in the following paragraphs.

Activation of Macrophages as a key Mechanism for *Tinospora cordifolia*

To demonstrate this, a rise in WBC count and neutrophilia were taken as parameters reflecting its nonspecific immunostimulatory activity.

Lipofundin S 20%, a stable soyabean preparation, was chosen as a macrophage blocker. Lipofundin S *per se* did not alter the WBC count but a decrease in the phagocytic activity of macrophages was noted ($25.75 \pm 10.82\%$ as compared to $31.33 \pm 1.15\%$ in normal rats, $p < 0.05$).

The effect of *Tinospora cordifolia* on WBC count and % neutrophils was studied in presence and absence of Lipofundin S. Rats were administered *Tinospora cordifolia* in the dose of 100 mg twice a day for 7 days. The leucocyte count was done basally (day 0) and repeated on day 7. The macrophage activity was assessed on day 7 using *Staphylococcus aureus* as the test organism. The total WBC counts on the 7th day of therapy with *Tinospora cordifolia* were significantly higher (WBC: $13250 \pm 2491.48/\text{mm}^3$, neutrophils $59 \pm 1.73\%$) than on day 0 (WBC count: $8066.66 \pm 659.96/\text{mm}^3$, neutrophils $46.5 \pm 4.23\%$ $p < 0.001$ vs day 7). The % phagocytosis of macrophages was significantly increased ($50.5 \pm 1.11\%$ vs $31.33 \pm 1.15\%$ in normal; $p < 0.001$).

When Lipofundin S was given concurrently with *Tinospora cordifolia* during this period, the rise in WBC count and neutrophils was inhibited ($7066.6 \pm 1556.34/\text{mm}^3$, $41 \pm 1.63\%$ respectively; $p < 0.01$) with associated decrease in phagocytic activity of macrophages ($37.16 \pm 6.06\%$) as compared to with *Tinospora cordifolia* alone. *Tinospora cordifolia* could not exhibit its nonspecific immunostimulant activity when macrophage function was blocked. In other words, activation of macrophages was essential for the immunostimulant effects of *Tinospora cordifolia* [23].

Link Between Immunostimulation and Differential Effect on Liver Damage

The first step in this direction was to determine the effect of macrophage activation on the structure and function of the liver. For this purpose, a model system established by Ferluga and Allison (1978) [24] was used. Activity of peritoneal macrophages was taken as a marker of immunostimulation.

Mice treated with *Tinospora cordifolia* for 14 days showed increased phagocytosis and killing by peritoneal macrophages but no change was detected in liver structure or function. Injection of an innocuous dose of lipopolysaccharide (25 µg) to animals pretreated with *Tinospora cordifolia* resulted in rise in serum AST and ALT levels, depletion of liver glycogen, necrosis of hepatocytes and mortality in 50% of animals. The activation of macrophages persisted. *Corynebacterium parvum*, a known immunostimulant, was taken as a positive control in this model, which also showed high mortality with necrosis. Thus, pretreatment with immunostimulants appears to activate macrophages and these activated macrophages on stimulation cause damage to the liver through their secretory products.

The findings of this experiment explain the results of our earlier studies [21–23] in which pretreatment with *Tinospora cordifolia* was found to potentiate the effects of hepatotoxins like CCl_4 or d-galactosamine. The macrophages activated by *Tinospora cordifolia* appear to liberate excess of cytotoxic products in response to toxin-induced necrosis. These products damage additional hepatocytes, thus potentiating damage.

Mononulear phagocytic activity and the effect of *Tinospora cordifolia* on it were also evaluated in models of chronic liver damage. The models selected were based on three different mechanisms of liver damage. These include free radicals [25], immune complexes [26] and obstruction to biliary duct [27]. A system was evolved to quantify the fibrotic deposition using ocular micrometry. This parameter was supported by a biochemical marker of fibrosis, hydroxyproline. Both phagocytic and killing activities of peritoneal macrophages were studied [28, 29]. Serum opsonin activity was also determined.

Therapy with *Tinospora cordifolia* was started after induction of chronic liver injury. All the abovementioned parameters were assessed following four weeks of treatment and compared with those from an untreated control group.

In all the three models, deposition of fibrosis was associated with altered phagocytic and killing activity of macrophages as well as changes in serum opsonin activity. *Tinospora cordifolia* effectively decreased the fibrous tissue depostion—more so in cirrhosis due to free radical injury. The drug therapy also normalised the activity of peritoneal macrophages. Opsonisation capacity of the serum was also found to improve.

Thus, the differential activity of *Tinospora cordifolia* was found to be related to its immunostimulant effect. Based on these findings, this agent can be a rational choice for chronic liver disorders like alcoholic or post-hepatitic cirrhosis, cholestasis and chronic active hepatitis which are characterised by fibrosis and immunosuppression.

Though peritoneal macrophages are of the same lineage as Kupffer cells and hence were selected as representative of the latter cells in earlier experiments, functional differences exist between the two elements [15]. Hence the next experiments were planned to study the function of Kupffer cells in chronic liver damage and the effect of *Tinospora cordifolia* was evaluated with respect to Kupffer cell activity.

Modulation of Kupffer Cell Activity

Initially, clearance of particulate matter (colloidal carbon) was studied in all the three models of chronic liver damage (induced by carbon tetrachloride, horse serum and bile duct ligation and sectioning). Prolongation of half-life of elimination of colloidal carbon was observed in chronic liver damage induced by either of the procedures.

After induction of damage, the rats were given either distilled water or *Tinospora cordifolia* and observed for a further period of 4 weeks (one week in a model of cholestasis). In all the three models, *Tinospora cordifolia*, was found to hasten the clearance of colloidal carbon as compared to the control group receiving distilled water. This suggests that therapy with *Tinospora cordifolia* improves the depressed phagocytic activity of Kupffer cells, the resident macrophages of the liver. A point to note was that the phagocytic function of Kupffer cells was improved by the drug despite the persistence of damaging mechanisms (immune complexes in horse serum-induced model and irreversible cholestasis after sectioning of the ligated duct) [23, 30, 31].

Though Kupffer cells constitute 2/3rd of total RES [32] other elements of the RES (peritoneal and alveolar macrophages) also take part in the clearance of carbon. Another experiment was planned in which an unique function of Kupffer cells, viz. uptake and processing of endotoxin [15] was studied. Kupffer cells serve as an efficient filtering mechanism for gut-related endotoxin and prevent their access to the systemic circulation [33]. Detection of endotoxin in the circulation therefore serves as a parameter to determine functional status of Kupffer cells.

Hence, to get a conclusive proof of activation of Kupffer cells, a bioassay was planned to detect endotoxins in circulation [34] in a model of cholestasis. This was based on the principle that rats with endotoxaemia are highly susceptible to injected lead acetate. The dose of lead acetate (7.5 mg/kg) that produces no effect in normal rats can induce mortality in animals having even picograms of endotoxins circulating in the body. The incidence of endotoxaemia was found to be higher in cholestatic rats (73.3%). Pretreatment with *Tinospora cordifolia* decreased this incidence significantly—especially when started early in the course of cholestasis (from day 1 of ligation, a group where only 30% mortality was encountered; $p < 0.05$).

Another way of detecting endotoxaemia is to study its biological effects. Sepsis, deranged haemostasis and exacerbation of ischaemic renal injury are the three characteristic effects of endotoxaemia [35, 36]. They also account for the complications observed in cholestasis [37]. In a model of cholestasis, the effect of *Tinospora cordifolia* was evaluated against these biological manifestations of endotoxaemia.

Tinospora cordifolia was found to offer protection against induced infection. The bacteraemia was reduced [38, 39]. It was also found to decrease the prolonged prothrombin time and even normalize it when given concurrently with vitamin K. It corrected the raised FDP/fibrinogen ratio [40], an adverse prognostic predictor of intravascular coagulation [41]. *Tinospora cordifolia* also reduced the rise in blood urea nitrogen, tubular necrosis and mortality which occurred following renal ischaemia in cholestasis [42].

Thus, *Tinospora cordifolia* was found to improve the impaired function of Kupffer cells in chronic liver damage as seen from increased uptake of particulate matter, and reduced spillover of endotoxin to circulation. It is also effective in preventing complications secondary to endotoxaemia.

Whether modulation of Kupffer cells occurs directly or indirectly by influencing extracellular matrix remains to be answered. Further work using biochemical markers of extracellular matrix and cytokines can shed light on the mechanism of action of *Tinospora cordifolia*.

This drug is widely used by Ayurvedic physicians. As mentioned earlier, it is also an ingredient of various multiherbal 'hepatoprotective' formulations available in the market. These formulations are commonly prescribed even by the practitioners of modern medicine. Hence, it was felt necessary to evaluate the effects of *Tinospora cordifolia* in clinical setting designing controlled clinical trials. This would help physicians to make a rational choice based on scientific proofs.

Clinical Studies

Tinospora cordifolia has been developed into a standardized formulation which contains whole aqueous extract prepared from powdered stems. The route of administration is oral. Phase 1 study carried out in normal volunteers to evaluate safety did not reveal any alterations in biochemical, immunological or radiological parameters.

Hepatic disorders with evidence of fibrosis and immunosuppression (viz. obstructive jaundice, asymptomatic carriers of hepatitis B antigen and cirrhosis) were selected to evaluate effects of *Tinospora cordifolia*. In all the three conditions, defect in Kupffer cell activity or mononuclear phagocyte activity has been reported [15, 39, 43]. Knowing the difficulties in assessment of fibrosis in humans, we monitored clinical signs and symptoms, complications and quality of life in these patients. To judge immunostimulation, activity of immune cells in terms of phagocytosis and killing capactiy was assessed.

Obstructive Jaundice

Maximum clinical exploration was done in patients with obstructive jaundice. Present pre-operative therapy aims only at decompression of the biliary tract, control of infection with antibiotics and vitamin K if there is a disturbance in haemostasis. Despite the improvements in peri-operative care, the surgical outcome of these patients has remained poor [44, 45]. Endotoxaemia resulting from depressed Kupffer cell activity is a well known feature of obstructive jaundice [37]. This is responsible for various complications including sepsis, renal failure, haemorrhages and disseminated intravascular coagulation observed in the patients [37, 46]. Based on the studies done in cholestatic rats it was felt that *Tinospora cordifolia* can be included in the therapeutic armamentarium of extrahepatic biliary obstruction.

We used *Tinospora cordifolia* as an add-on regime to conventional therapy. The two groups of patients were well matched with respect to clinical features, hepatic and immune functions. The neutrophil activity of these patients was significantly lower as compared to normal healthy donors. Following biliary drainage bactobilia was observed. Therapy with *Tinospora cordifolia* significantly decreased the mortality from 92% to 40%. This was associated with decrease in septicaemia. *Tinospora cordifolia* was found to potentiate the depressed neutrophil activity [47]. This corroborates our findings in animals. Later, a randomized, double blind, placebo controlled study was planned with a single surgical unit, the results of which also showed significant reduction in mortality rates. This drug is now being routinely prescribed to all patients with obstructive jaundice attending our GI surgical unit.

Recently we carried out an assay for serum GMCSF levels in 12 patients before and after therapy with *Tinospora cordifolia*. Mononuclear cells were separated by Ficoll Hypaque density gradient centrifugation from human umbilical cord blood and were seeded on methyl cellulose agar as progenitor cells responding to colony stimulating factors present in the serum. Using this soft agar assay [48] the number of GM colonies formed on the 14th day were counted. Number of colonies was found to increase following therapy (54.50 ± 25.89 on day 10 vs 35.70 ± 20.89 before therapy; $p < 0.05$). The neutrophils of these patients also showed an increase in phagocytic activity ($34.64 \pm 8.15\%$ vs $29.82 \pm 5.92\%$; $p < 0.05$).

Patients with obstructive jaundice often show high morbidity which is related to poor hepatobiliary function and the complications present. This contributes to poor quality of life. The patients treated with *Tinospora cordifolia* expressed a feeling of well being, their appetite improved, and none of them required postponement of surgery because of complications. No side effects have been detected with *Tinospora cordifolia*.

As fullness of stomach and feeling of bloated abdomen were common complaints from the patients with obstructive jaundice, in some of these patients (n = 10) we determined orocaecal transit time. This time reflects the changes in gastrointestinal motility. In obstructive jaundice gastrointestinal motility was found to be reduced, prolonging the transit time (9.35 ± 2.37 hrs vs 5.85 ± 1.7 hrs in normal; $p < 0.005$). However the patients treated with *Tinospora cordifolia* revealed normalization of GI transit time (6.20 ± 2.19 hrs). This additional effect, unrelated to immunostimulation, may also be contributing to the improvement in quality of life observed in pateints with *Tinospora cordifolia*.

Asymptomatic Carriers of HBsAg

In asymptomatic carriers of HBsAg, elimination of viral antigen is necessary to prevent future hepatic dysfuntion and to reduce transmission. Though the role of nonspecific cellular immunity is not clearly defined, defects in monocyte functions have been reported [49–51] and immunomodulators like levamisole, cyanidanol and interferons have been shown to eliminate antigen [52–54]. We therefore selected carriers from the blood donors list available in the blood bank who were allocated randomly to 2 treatment groups—placebo or *Tinospora cordifolia* (16 mg/kg/day). Therapy was given for 2 months. Seroconversion of HBsAg status was looked for along with monocyte functions.

In asymptomatic carriers of hepatitis B, therapy with *Tinospora cordifolia* for 2 months led to seroconversion in 37.5% of patients. This rate was 3 times higher than that observed in the placebo group. In all the patients who showed seroconversion, improvement was observed in the intracellular killing capacity of monocytes ($51.67 \pm 6.5\%$) as compared to that in the placebo group ($38.38 \pm 12.06\%$). This trend towards elimination of viral antigen needs to be investigated further especially in pateints with chronic active hepatitis.

Cirrhosis

Cirrhosis is yet another disease in which suppression of Kupffer cell activity is well documented [15]. In an earlier study conducted by us a significant depression of phagocytic and killing capacity of monocytes ($20.58 \pm 5\%$ phago and $41.24 \pm 12.9\%$ ICK) was observed in cirrhotics as compared to normal volunteers ($27.89 \pm 3.63\%$ phago and $50.91 \pm 6.3\%$ ICK, n = 50) [29]. Defects in monocyte phagocytosis and intracellular killing capacity as well as in serum opsonin activity have been reported by other research workers [43, 55].

A preliminary study was planned to judge whether *Tinospora cordifolia* has any beneficial effect on the course of disease in 12 patients with moderate cirrhosis. The patients were randomly allocated to 2 groups. Both the groups were matching with respect to metabolic capacity of liver (a quantitative liver function which predicts prognosis). This showed that prognosis in these two groups was identical. One group received *Tinospora cordifolia* and the other placebo for a period of 6 months.

The clinico-biochemical findings were graded to get a composite score using Child-Pugh system and monitored monthly for 6 months. Incidence of complications, metabolic capacity of liver (as determined by estimation of antipyrine half-life), assessment of monocyte activity and serum defect were the other parameters monitored during the 6 months of follow up.

At the end of this period, 1 patient from the placebo group showed improvement, 2 remained static while 3 worsened. In the group treated with

Tinospora cordifolia, 4 patients showed improvement. This difference was also reflected in change in metabolic capacity of the liver. In the placebo group there was a slow, progressive worsening (Antipyrine half-life increased from 16.6 ± 5.6 hrs to 19.27 ± 3.78 hrs) while in the group treated with *Tinospora cordifolia* there was a significant shortening of antipyrine half-life (16.24 ± 4.2 hrs to 14.5 ± 3.9 hrs; $p < 0.05$).

The % phagocytosis and killing capacity of monocytes in both the groups were comparable at the start of the trial (Phago: $23.4 \pm 5.68\%$ and $18.5 \pm 5.86\%$ and ICK: $38.36 \pm 4.8\%$ and $35.31 \pm 8.82\%$ respectively) and were significantly lower than normal (Phago: $27.89 \pm 3.63\%$ and ICK: $50.91 \pm 6.3\%$; n = 50). However at the end of follow-up, a significant improvement occurred in the *Tinospora cordifolia*-treated group (Phago: $40.3 \pm 3.2\%$ and ICK: $45.81 \pm 5.5\%$). The values of % phgocytosis were significantly higher than normal. No change was found in the placebo group (Phago: $21.5 \pm 4.95\%$ and ICK: $37.5 \pm 3.54\%$).

To find out serum opsonin activity, monocytes of normal volunteers were incubated with sera samples from the same volunteer, i.e. autologous control and also with test sera from patients receiving either *Tinospora cordifolia* or placebo. Any deviation in the activity of normal monocytes under the influence of test sera reflected the defect in opsonization capacity.

The phagocytic activity of the monocytes was found to be reduced when incubated with sera from cirrhotic patients; however the difference was not significant when compared to the paired control. Intracellular killing capacity of these cells was also found to be significantly decreased ($39.81 \pm 7.1\%$ vs $54.08 \pm 5.9\%$ and $39.9 \pm 4.8\%$ vs $51.28 \pm 6.1\%$ in autologous control; $p < 0.01$).

After 3 months of therapy with *Tinospora cordifolia*, the sera samples were collected and incubated with normal monocytes. At this time no deviation was observed in phagocytosis and intracellular killing of these cells ($49.87 \pm 4.7\%$) as compared to autologous controls ($52.26 \pm 3.6\%$). In the patients receiving placebo, ICK values ($41.67 \pm 5.76\%$) remained lower than the autologous control ($55.22 \pm 3.3\%$; $p < 0.05$). Same was the status at the end of 6 months.

Thus in cirrhotics, therapy with *Tinospora cordifolia* improved immunological functions, metabolic capacity and Child-Pugh scores. Though this was a pilot study planned to judge the potential benefit of therapy, the positive findings demand a well designed controlled trial in larger patient population.

Conclusion

The data of the three clinical trials conducted by us provide a novel approach for therapy of liver disorders. In all the three conditions, having different etiologies and pathogenesis, the drug has proven its potential. Oral efficacy of this immunostimulant coupled with wide therapeutic range have provided a new weapon to physicians to fight against uncontrolled fibrotic depositions in chronic liver diseases and other connective tissue disorders.

Acknowledgements

We are grateful to Merind Ltd. for manufacturing and supplying standardized whole aqueous extract of *Tinospora cordifolia*. We also acknowledge the encouragement from Dr. P.M. Pai, Director, ME & MH and Dean, Seth G.S. Medical College & KEM Hospital.

References

1. Charaka Samhita. Chikitsasthana. Chapter 6; Stanzas 7, 8. Sharma P. Ed. Varanasi: Chaukhambha Orientalia, 1983; 3–4.
2. Sushrut Samhita. Sootrasthana. Chapter 1; Stanza 7. Shastri AK Ed. Varanasi: Chaukhambha Orientalia, 1983; 3.
3. Katiyar C.K., Brindavanam N.B., Tiwari P., Narayana D.B.A., Immunomodulator products from Ayurveda: Current status and future perspectives. In: Upadhyay SN (Ed), Immunomodulation, New Delhi: Narosa Publishing House. 1997; 163–87.
4. Thatte U.M. and Dahanukar S.A. 1989. Immunotherapeutic modification of experimental infections by Indian Medicinal Plants. *Phytotherapy Res.* **3(2):** 43–49.
5. Patil M., Patki P., Kamath H.V., Patwardhan B. 1997. Antistress activity of *Tinospora cordifolia* (wild) Miers, *Indian Drugs* **34(4):** 211–215.
6. Atal C.K., Sharma M.L., Kaul A. and Khazuria A. 1986. Immunomodulating agents of plant origin. I: Preliminary screening, *J. Ethhnopharmacol.* **18:** 133–141.
7. Sainis K.B., Sumariwalla P.F., Goel A., Chintalwar G.J., Sipahimalani A.T., Banerji A. Immunomodulatory properties of stem extracts of *Tinospora cordifolia*: Cell targets and active principles. In: Upadhyay S.N. (Ed), Immunomodulation, New Delhi: Narosa Publishing House. 1997; 155–62.
8. Sherlock S. Hepatic transplantation. In: Diseases of the Liver and Biliary system. Oxford: Blackwell Sci. Publ, 1975; 550–6.
9. Lee W.M. Drug induced hepatotoxicity. *N. Eng. J. Med.* 1995; **333:** 1118–26.
10. Schuppan D., Somasundaram R., Just M. The extracellular matrix: a major signal transduction network. In: Clement B., Guillouzo A. Eds. Cellular and Molecular Aspects of Cirrhosis, Vol 216. Colloque INSERN/John Libbey Eurotext Ltd. 1992; 115–34.
11. Popper H. Regulatory modulation in hepatology. *Hepatology* 1987; **7:** 586–90.
12. Decker K. Eicosanoids, signal molecules of liver cell. *Semin. Liver Dis.* 1985; **5:** 175–90.
13. Shiratori Y., Kawase T., Shiina S., et al. Modulation of hepatotoxicity by macrophages in the liver. *Hepatology* 1988; **8:** 815–21.
14. Tsukamoto H., Gaal K., French S., Insights into the pathogenesis of alcoholic liver necrosis and fibrosis. status report. *Hepatology* 1990; **12:** 599–608.
15. Toth C.A., Thomas P., Liver endocytosis and Kupffer cells. *Hepatology* 1992; **16:** 255–66.
16. Charaka Samhita. Chikitsasthana. Chapter 6; Stanza 134. Sharma P. Ed. Varanasi: Chaukhambha Orientalia, 1983; 285.

17. Bhaishajaratnavali. Plehayakrutorgachikitsaprakaranam. Chapter 41; Stanza 12. Rajeshwardattashastri Ayurvedashastracharya. Ed. Varanasi: Chaukhamba Sanskrit Samsthan 1987; 542.
18. Nighantaratnakar. Gunadoshaprakarana. Javaji P. Ed. Mumbai: Nirnayasagar Press, 74.
19. Handa S.S., Sharma A., Chakraborti K.K. Natural products and plants as liver protecting drugs. *Fitoterapia* 1986; **LVII:** 307–50.
20. Bhaisharjaratnavali, 5: 429, 41: 59. Varanasi: Choukhamba Sanskrit Pustakalaya, 1951.
21. Rege N.N., Dahanukar S.A., Karandikar S.M. Hepatoprotective effect of *Tinospora cordifolia* against carbon tetrachloride induced liver damage. *Indian Drugs* 1984; **21:** 544–55.
22. Rege N.N., Dahanukar S.A., Karandikar S.M. Hepatoprotection by indigenous agents. The Indian Practitioner 1985; **38:** 551–6.
23. Rege N.N. Evaluation of hepatoprotective effect of Tinospora cordifolia. Ph. D. Thesis, University of Mumbai, Mumbai, 1996.
24. Ferluga J., Allison A.C. Role of mononuclear infiltrating cells in pathogenesis of hepatitis. *Lancet* 1978; **2:** 610–11.
25. Chen T.S., Chen P.J. Hepatic fibrosis and cirrhosis. In: Essential Hepatology. London: Butterworth Co Publ, 1977; 155–62.
26. Paronetto F., Popper H. Chronic liver injury induced by immunological reactions. *Am. J. Pathol.* 1996; **49:** 1087–1101.
27. Cameron G.R., Oakley C.L. Ligation of the common bile duct. *J. Pathol. Bacteriol.* 1932; **35:** 769–98.
28. Lehrer R.I. Measurement of candidacidal activity of specific leucocyte types in mixed cell populations. *Infect. Immun.* 1970; **20:** 42–7.
29. Rege N.N., Dahanukar S.A. Quantitation of microbicidal activity of mononuclear phagocytes: *an in vitro* technique. *J. Postgrad. Med.* 1993; **39:** 22–5.
30. Nagarkatti D.S., Rege N.N., Desai N.K., Dahanukar S.A. Modulation of Kupffer cell activity by Tinospora cordifolia in liver damage. *J. Postgrad. Med.* 1994; **40:** 65–67.
31. Malgi S. Modulation of Liver Injury by Plant Products. Thesis for M.Sc. (Applied Biology), University of Mumbai, Mumbai, 1989.
32. Saba T.M. Physiology and pathophysiology of reticulonendothelial system. *Arch. Intern. Med.* 1970; **126:** 1031–52.
33. Nolan J.P., Camara D.S. Endotoxin and liver disease. In: Knook D.L., Wisse E. Eds. Sinusoidal Liver Cells. Amsterdam: Elsevier Biomed Press, 1982; 377–86.
34. Filkins J.P. Bioassay of endotoxin inactivation in the lead sensitized rat. *Proc. Soc. Exp. Biol. Med.* 1970; **134:** 610–12.
35. Nolan J.P. Endotoxin, reticuloendothelial function and liver injury. *Hepatology* 1981; **1:** 458–65.
36. Bourgoignie J.J., Valle G.A. Endotoxin and renal dysfunction in liver disease. In: Epstein M. Ed. The Kidney in Liver Disease, 3rd ed. Baltimore: Williams and Wilkins, 1988; 486–502.
37. Greve J.W. Complications in obstructive jaundice. An experimental study on etiology and prevention. Ph.D. Thesis, University of Limburg, Maastricht, 1990.
38. Rege N.N., Malagi S.P., More P.B., Nazareth H.M., Bapat R.D., Karandikar S.M., Dahanukar S.A. Immunostimulant effect of *Tinospora cordifolia* in experimental surgical jaundice (A). *J. Gastroenterol. Hepatol.* 1988; **3:** 546.
39. Rege N.N., Nazareth H.M., Bapat R.D., Dahanukar S.A. Modulation of immunosuppression in obstructive jaundice by *Tinospora cordifolia. Indian J. Med. Res.*1989; **90:** 478–83.

40. Javale H.S. Haemorrhagic complications in obstructive jaundice and its modulation by *Tinospora cordifolia*. Thesis for M.Sc. (Applied Biology), University of Mumbai, Mumbai, 1994.

41. Allison M.E.M., Prentice C.R.M., Kennedy A.C., Blumgart L.H. Renal function and other factors in obstructive jaundice. *Br. J. Surg.* 1979; **66:** 392–7.

42. Dahanukar S.A., Rege N.N., Koti R., Bapat R.D. Antiendotoxaemic effect of *Tinospora cordifolia* (S68). Abstract Book of Inaugural World Congress of the International Hepato-Pancreato-Biliary Association, May 31-June 3, 1994, Boston, p. 36.

43. Hassner A., Kletter Y., Shlag D., Yedvab M., Aronson M., Shibolet S. Impaired monocyte function in cirrhosis. *Br. Med. J.* 1981; **282:** 1263–3.

44. Dixon J.M., Armstrong C.P., Duffy S.W., Davies G.C. Factors affecting morbidity and mortality after surgery for obstructive jaundice: a review of 373 patients. *Gut* 1983; **24:** 845–52.

45. Greig J.D., Krukowski Z.H., Matheson N.A. Surgical morbidity and mortality in one hundred and twenty-nine patients with obstructive jaundice. *Br. J. Surg.* 1988; **75:** 216–9.

46. Drives G., James O., Wardie N., Study of reticuloendothelial phagocytic activity in patients with cholestasis. *Br. Med. J.* 1976; **1:** 1568–9.

47. Rege N.N., Bapat R.D., Koti R., Desai N.K., Dahanukar S.A. Immunotherapy with Tinospora cordifolia: A new lead in the management of obstructive jaundice. *Indian J. Gastroenterol.* 1993; **12(1):** 5–8.

48. Hows J.M., Bradley B.A., march J.C.W., et al. Growth of human umbilical cord blood in longterm haemopoietic cultines. *Lancet* 1992; **340:** 73–6.

49. Dudley F.J., Fax R.A., Sherlock S. Cellular immunity and hepatitis associated Australia antigen liver disease. *Lancet* 1972; **1:** 723–6.

50. Rege N., Abraham P., Kulkarni M., Desai N.K., Ray V., Dahanukar S.A. Monocyte function in asymptomatic carriers of hepatitis B surface antigen (A). *Indian J. Gastroenterol.* 1989; **8:** A38.

51. Alberty A.G., Realdi G., Bortolotti F., Rigoletti A.M. T lymphocyte cytotoxicity to HBsAg coated target cells inhepatitis B infection. *Gut* 1977; **18:** 1004–9.

52. Greenberg H.B., Pollard R.B., Lutwick L.I., Gregory P.B., Robinson W.S., Merigan T.C. Effect of human leucocyte interferon on hepatitis B virus infection in patients with chronic active hepatitis. *N. Eng. J. Med.* 1976; **295:** 517–22.

53. Par A., Barma K., Hollots I., et al. Levamisole in viral hepatitis. *Lancet* 1977; **I:** 702.

54. Vallotton J., Frei P.C. Influence of (±) cyanidanol-3 on the leucocyte migration inhibition test carried out in the presence of purified protein derivative and hepatitis B surface antigen. *Infect. Immun.* 1981; **32:** 432–7.

55. Holdstock G., Leslie B., Hill S., Tanner A.R.,Wright R., Monocyte function in cirrohosis. *J. Clin. Pathol.* 1982; **35:** 972–9.

Immunopharmacology: Strategies for immunotherapy
S.N. Upadhyay (Ed)

12. Cross-Linking Activating and Inhibitory Immunoreceptors: A novel mechanism of immunosuppression

Wolf H. Fridman

INSERM U255, Immunologie Cellulaire et Clinique, Institut Curie, Paris, France

Summary

First demonstrated on B lymphocytes, where the cross-linking of the B cell receptor (BCR) to the Fcγ Receptor (FcγR) by anti BCR antibodies results in inhibition of B cell activation, the concept of the inhibitory function of the type IIB FcγR (FcγR IIb) was extended to cross-linking with the T cell receptor (TCR), the high affinity IgE receptor (FcεRI) and the activating Fcγ Receptors (FcγR I, FcγR III and FcγR IIa). A tyrosine-based inhibitory motif (ITIM) was identified and shown to be tyrosine-phosphorylated following aggregation of the activating receptor and tyrosine kinase engagement. Phosphorylated ITIM then bind an SH2-inositol phosphatase (SHIP) resulting in inhibition of Ca^{++} influx.

Other receptors with inhibitory function, as well as a large family of molecules which regulate cell activation have been shown to possess ITIMs. Among these receptors Killer Inhibitory Receptors on NK and T cells, CTLA-4 on T cells and CD22 on B cells negatively regulate NK, T and B cell activation. They act by a mechanism slightly different than FcγR, being tyrosine-phosphorylated upon their own aggregation and then binding different SH2-phosphatases, such as SHP-1 and SHP-2 which act on the phosphotyrosines of downstream effectors of the ITAM sequence of the activating TCR or FcR.

A general mechanism of regulation of cell activation in the immune system arises from the interaction between activating and inhibitory immunoreceptors, by using consensus ITIM sequences, but different pathways of phosphatase-mediated cell inactivation.

Activating Immunoreceptors

All cells participating in a immune response can interact, directly or indirectly, with antigen. For this purpose, B and T lymphocytes are equipped with receptors which directly bind antigen in its native form or when presented by Major Histocompatibility Complex (MHC) molecules, respectively. The B cell Receptor (BCR) is composed of a membrane Immunoglobulin (Ig) which binds antigen, associated to dimers of non antigen-binding transmembrane chains, called Igα and Igβ Fig. 1. Similarly, the T cell Receptor (TCR) is made of an antigen-binding unit (TCRαβ or TCRγδ), associated to non antigen-binding transmembrane elements composing the CD3 complex (CD3δ, ε, γ, ζ). In both receptors, the antigen-binding units are apparently devoid of any signalling potential, they serve as specificity ensuring elements that will initiate immune reactions. In contrast, their associated chains bear consensus motifs which trigger cell activation. These motifs are composed of two YxxL sequences (where Y is a tyrosine and L a leucin, and x any amino acid) separated by an average of 7 amino acids (Fig. 1). The mechanism by which cells are triggered by these receptors is similar. First, the binding of the antigen recognition units to multivalent antigens aggregate the receptors resulting in the phosphorylation, by an SH2-containing proteine tyrosine kinase of the src family (lyn, fyn, lck...) of the tyrosines present in the signalling units

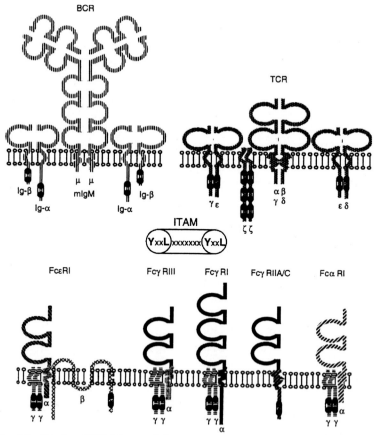

Fig. 1. The family of ITAM-containing receptors: BCR: B cell Receptor : TCR: T cell Receptor: FcR: Fc Receptor: ITAM: Immunoreceptor Tyrosine-based Activation Motif.

of the receptors. The two phosphorylated tyrosines of the activating motifs then bind SH2-containing protein tyrosine kinases of the syk family (syk in B cells, zap 70 in T cells) which initiate various activation pathways, via PLCγ mobilisation leading to Ca^{++} in flux, via P13 kinase phosphorylation or via the Ras pathway, eventually leading to the transcription of cytokine genes and cell proliferation [1, 2]. Figure 2 illustrate, with the times in which each step takes place, this pathway in B lymphocytes.

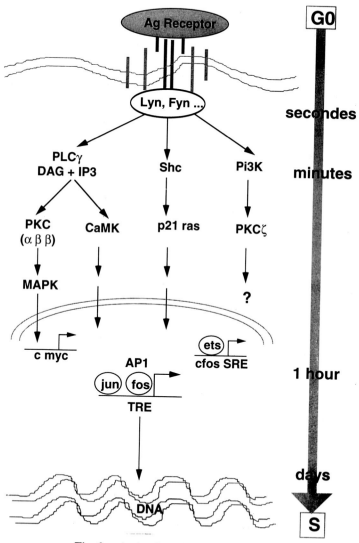

Fig. 2. Activation of B lymphocytes.

Immunocompetent cells other than B and T lymphocytes also interact with antigen. However, their interaction is indirect, via the binding of antibody-associated molecules. These cells bear receptors for the Fc region of immunoglobulins, i.e. Fc Receptors (FcR). FcR for all Ig isotypes, but IgM, have been molecularly characterized. With the exeption of low affinity receptors for IgE and IgD which belong to the family of animal lectins, all FcR are members of the Ig superfamily, as the BCR and the TCR [3]. Some Fc receptors trigger cell activation. For instance high affinity IgE receptors (FcεRI) induce the release of inflammatory mediators by mast cells and basophils. High affinity IgG receptors (FCγRI) and IgA receptors (FcαR) trigger an oxygen burst in macrophages and myeloïd cells, while low affinity IgG receptors (FcγRIII) are responsible for the antibody dependent cell cytotoxicity (ADCC) exerted by NK cells and macrophages [4]. These various cell-activating Fc receptors are built on the same model as the BCR and the TCR. They have a ligand-binding subunit, called the α chain, which specifically interacts with IgE, IgA or IgG, respectively and is associated with non-Ig binding signal transducing chains, which bear a signalling motif, similar to that of the BCR and TCR associated chains (Fig. 1). One exception is forwarded by an human low affinity IgG receptor (FcαRIIA/C) in which the signalling motif is borne by the intracellular region of the IgG-binding chain. For the other receptors, the triggering unit is composed either by an homodimer of γ chains (in macrophages and murine NK cells), or an heterodimer of γ and ζ chains (in human NK cells) or an heterodimer of γ and β chains (in mast cells) [3]. The mechanism of activation used by FcR is similar to that used by BCR and TCR. Thus, the aggregation of FcR molecules, by and antigen-bound immunoglobulins, results in the phosphorylation of intracellular tyrosines by protein tyrosine kinase of the src family (lyn or fyn), followed by the binding of syk to these phosphorylated tyrosines and down stream cell activation [5].

All the receptors, members of the Ig superfamily, reacting directly or indirectly with antigen have been named immunoreceptors and the tyrosine-based activating motifs present in these receptors are thus called Immunoreceptor Tyrosine-based Activation Motifs (ITAM). Table I depict these motif, including similar sequences strinkingly found on lymphotropic activating viruses [6]. Figure 3 illustrates the general way by which ITAM-containing receptors trigger cell activation [5, 7].

Inhibitory Immunoreceptors

Physiological mechanisms control immune responses, either by terminating immune reactions or by forbidding their initiation and development.

An example of immune reaction termination is provided by the negative feed-back exerted by IgG antibodies on their own production. It has been known for a long time that the injection of minute amounts of IgG antibodies terminates antibody production in mouse and that it requires an intact Fc region [8]. A possible mechanism for this inhibition follows from "in vitro" experiments showing that the cross-linking, by IgG antibodies, of the b cell receptor and Fcγ receptors inhibits cell activation. The molecular analysis of

Table 1. Immunoreceptor Tyrosine-based activation motifs (ITAM)

hζ1	N Q L Y N E L N L G R R E E	Y D V L
hζ2	E G L Y N E L Q K D K M A E A	Y S E I
hζ3	D G L Y D G L S T A T K D T	Y D A L
CD3γ	D Q L Y D P L K D R E D D Q	Y S H L
CD3δ	D Q V Y Q P L R D R D D A Q	Y S H L
CD3ε	N P D Y E P I T K G Q R D L	Y S G L
Igα	E N L Y E G L N L D D C S M	Y E D I
Igβ	D H T Y E G L N I D Q T A T	Y E D I
rFcεR1 γ	D A V Y T G L N T R N Q E T	Y E T L
rFcεR1 β	D R L Y E E L H V W S P I	Y S A L
EBV-LMP2A	P E I Y S H L S P V K P D	Y I N L
BLV gp130	D S D Y Q A L L P S A P E I	Y S H L
Consensus	D X X Y X X L X X X X X X X X X	Y X X L
	E I	I

the B cell FcγR revealed that it is composed of a single chain, devoid of ITAM sequences, but bearing, in its intracytoplasmic region, a tyrosine-containing motif required for cell inhibition [9]. Further analysis in other cells of the immune system demonstrated that this particular FcγR, called FcγRIIb, inhibits signalling through all ITAM-containing immunoreceptors,

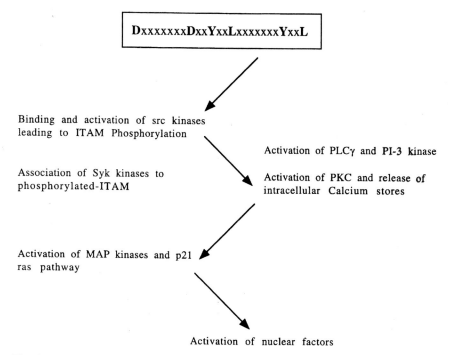

Fig. 3. **Cascade of signal transduction through ITAM clustering: ITAM: Immunoreceptor Tyrosine-based Activation Motif: PLC: Phospholipase C: PI-3: Phosphatydil inositol-3: MAP: Mitogen Activated Protein.**

i.e. the BCR, the TCR and the activating FcR, such as FcγRI, FcγRIIa... [10]. Since the tyrosine was an absolute requirement for inhibition to take place, the acronym ITIM, for Immunoreceptor Tyrosine Inhibitory Motif, was proposed for the inhibitory sequence [10].

It soon became evident that other molecules than FcγRIIb contained ITIM sequences. Strikingly, they all are involved in cell control, mostly in negative regulation of cell activation [7]. Among these are receptors that negatively signal in NK cells and T cells. Killer inhibitory receptors recognize self MHC class I molecules and present NK cells to destroy autologous MHC class I positive cells [11]. CTLA-4 bind B7 molecules on target cells and compete with CD28 in the regulation of T cell activation. Other ITIM containing receptors inhibit mast cell activation [12]. Table 2 depict the growing family of ITIM-containing receptors [13]. The mechanisms by which ITIM control cell activation mirrors that of ITAMs. The first step requires aggregation of the inhibitory receptor followed by phosphorylation of the tyrosine in the inhibitory motif. Different strategies are, however used by different ITIM-containing receptors. The homo aggregation of KIR and CTLA-4 is sufficient

Table 2. **Immunoreceptor Tyrosine-based Inhibition Motifs (ITIM) sequences of negative coreceptors**

IgSF members

mFcγRIIB	dleeaakteaentItyslLkhpealdeete-	
hFcγRIIB	npdeadkvgaentItYslLmhpdaleepdd- -	
hKIR	p58.183.N	vnredsdeqdpqeVtYaqLnhevftgrkit - -
hKIR	p58.183.C	rpsqrpktpptdiIvYteLpnaep - - - - - - - -
hKIR	p58. EB6.N	ansedsdeqdpqeVtYtqLnhcvftqrkit - -
hKIR	p58.EB6.C	rpsqrpktpptdiIvYteLpnaesrskvvscp
hKIR	p70.N	ansedsdeqdpeeVtYaqLdhcvftqrkit - -
hKIR	p70.C	rpsqrpktpptdtIlYteLpnakprskvvs - -
h CD22. 2	hslgcynpmmedgIsYttLrfpemniprtgda	
hCD22. 5	yenvipdfpedegIhYseLiqfgvge - - - - - -	
hCD22. 6	- - - - - - rpqaqenVdYviLkh - - - - - - - - - -	
mCD22. 2	qsqgcynpamddtVsYaiLrfpesdthnagda	
mCD22. 5	yenvnpscpedesIhYseLvqfgagk - - - - - -	
mCD22. 6	- - - - - - rpqakedVdYvtLkh - - - - - - - - - -	
mCTLA-4	- - - - - kkrsplttGvYvkMpptepecekfqp	
hCTLA-4	- - - - - kkrsplttGvYvkMpptepecekqfqp	
gp49B1.N	lnswnpqnedpqIvYaqVkpsrlqkdtacke	
gp 49B1. C	rlqkdtacketqdVtYaqLcirtqeqnns	

Type-C lectins

mKIR	Ly49A	- - - - - - - mseqeVtYsmVrfhksaglqkq- -
mKIR	Ly49C	- - - - - - - mseqeVtYttLrfhkssglqnp- -
mKIR	Ly49G4	- - - - - - - mseqeVtYstVrfhessrlqkl- -
NKG2A.N	- - - - - - - - mdnqgViYsdLnlppnpkrqqr - -	
NKG2A.C	kgnkssilateqeItYaeLnlqkasqdfqg- -	
MAFA	- - - - - - - - - madnSiYstLelpaaprvqddsr	

to activate the receptor-linked scr kinases which phosphorylate the ITIM tyrosine. For FcγRIIb, a cross-linking to the activating receptor (BCR, TCR, FcϵRI...) is necessary in order to achieve phosphorylation of the ITIM by lyn associated to the activating receptor [14]. After being phosphorylated the tyrosine recruit SH2-containing phosphatases, an inositol phosphatase (SHIP) for FcγRIIB, or tyrosine phosphatases, SHP1 and SHP2, for KIR and CTLA-4, respectively [12]. The type of phosphatase mobilized illustrates the function of the different ITIM containing receptors, an early, rapid blockade of NK or T cell cytotoxicity requiring an early inhibitory effect by dephosphorylation of cystream tyrosine-containing mediators, such as PI3 kinase [13], while a late termination of antibody production by FcγRII being compatible with the mobilisation of a phosphatase (SHIP) interfering dowstream with the inositif phosphate synthesis (Fig. 4).

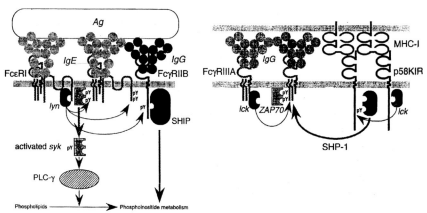

Fig. 4. **Two modes of action of ITIM-bearing receptors: FcR: Fc receptor: PLC: Phospholipase C:SHP: SH2-containing phosphatase: SHIP: SH2-containing inositol phosphatase: MHC: Major histocompatibility complex: KIR: Killer inhibitory receptor.**

Future Prospects

The elucidation of a general mechanism of control of cell activation paves the way for the conception of novel immunomodulatory molecules which would suppress immune responses by cross-linking ITAM and ITIM-containing immunoreceptors.

In addition, the concept should largely expand outside of the immune system since, on the one hand, ITAM and ITIM containing immunoreceptors are found ectopically expressed on non immunocompetent cells, particularly tumor cells, and on the other hand, molecules apparently unrelated to the immune system which bear ITIM being to be identified, opening the network of interactions to many cells in the organism.

References

1. Cambier J.C., Pleinman C.M., Clark M.R. Signal transducing by the B cell antigen receptor ant its co-receptors. *Annu. Rev. Immunol.,* 1994, **12**: 457–486.
2. Chan A.C., Desai D.M., Weiss A. The role of protein tyrosine kinases and protein tyrosine phosphatases in T cell antigen receptor signal transduction. *Annu. Rev. Immunol.,* 1994, **12**: 555–592.
3. Ravetch J.V., Kine J.P. Fc receptors. *Annu. Rev. Immunol.,* 1991, **9**: 457–492.
4. Fridman W.H., Sautès C. Cell-mediated effects of immunoglobulins. Ed. R.G. Landes Company, 1996, 1–201.
5. Bonnerot C. Cell activation via Fc receptors. In "Cell-mediated effects of immunoglobulins", ed. by Fridman W.H. and Sautès C. R.G. Landes Company, 67–88.
6. Reth M.G. Antigen receptor tail clue. *Nature,* 1989, **338**: 383–384.
7. Daëron M. Fc receptor biology. *Annu. Rev. Immunol.,* 1997, **15**: 203–234.
8. Sinclair N.R., St C., Chan P.L. Regulation of the immune response IV. The role of the Fc fragment in feedback inhibition by antibody. In: "Morphological and fundamental aspects of immunity" Plenum press, New York, 1971, 609–915.
9. Amigorena S., Bonnerot C., Drake J.R., Choquet D., Hunziker W., Guillet J.G., Webster P., Sautès C., Mellman I., Fridman W.H. Cytoplasmic domain heterogeneity and functions of IgG Fc receptors in B-lymphocytes. *Science,* 1992, **256**: 1808–1812.
10. Daëron M., Latour S., Malbec O., Espinosa E., Pina P., Pasmans S., Fridman W.H. The same tyrosine-based inhibition motif, in the intracytoplasmic domain of FcγRIIB, regulates negatively BCR-, TCR-, and FcR-dependent cell activation. *Immunity,* 1995, **6**: 635–646.
11. NK cells, MHC class I antigens and missing self. *Immunol. Rev.,* 1997, 155.
12. Vivier E., Daëron M. Immunoreceptor tyrosine-based inhibition motifs. *Immunol. Today,* 1997, in Press.
13. Cambier J.C. Inhibitory receptors abound? PNAS, 1997, 5993–5995.
14. Malbec O., Fong D.C., Turner M., Tybulewicz V.L., Cambier J.C., Fridman W.H., Daëron M. FcεRI- associated lyn-dependent phosphorylation of FcγRIIB during negative regulation of mast cell activation. *J. Immunol,* 1998, in Press.

Immunopharmacology: Strategies for immunotherapy
S.N. Upadhyay (Ed)

13. Immunomodulation of Murine Collagen-Induced Arthritis

C. Fournier*, G. Chiocchia*, N. Bessis*, A. Doncarli*, F. Batteux*, O. Abehsira-Amar* and M.C. Boissier*†

*INSERM U477, Université René Descartes, Hôpital Cochin, Paris, France

†Department of Rheumatology, Hôpital Avicenne, UFR Léonard de Vinci, Bobigny, France

Abstract

Polyarticular inflammation developing in collagen-induced arthritis (CIA) mimics the clinical and histological features of rheumatoid arthritis. CIA is acquired upon immunization with native type II collagen (CII) of susceptible strains of mice (DBA/1) and accumulating evidence during the past decade demonstrated the pivotal role of T cells in the initiation and the perpetuation of the disease. Thus, counteracting the effect of autoimmunity in CIA can be achieved by approaches targeting on autoaggressive T cells.

In this context, we have previously shown that vaccination with CII-specific T cell hybridomas (of either CD4 or CD8 phenotype) was effective in preventing the development of arthritis and even reverse the ongoing inflammation. More recently, we provided arguments indicating that CD4+ T cells expressing the Th1 phenotype are crucial initiators of the response. Furthermore, we have isolated and characterized a recurrent CD4+ T cell clone recognizing the immunodominant determinant of CII. Interestingly, when inoculated into DBA/1 mice, this clone exacerbates the severity of CIA.

On the other hand, we found that CII-specific Th2 cells develop later in the time course of the experimental disease and may contribute to the spontaneous remission of the pathology. Indeed, preventive administration of IL-4 or IL-13, by a powerful strategy of cellular gene therapy, reduced the arthritic process in CIA. Experiments using TNF-α transgenic mice revealed that one of the mechanisms underlying the beneficial effect of these Th2 cytokines may depend on the downregulation of proinflammatory cytokines (TNF-α and IL-1).

Since the cellular gene therapy that we used was based on the engraftment of chinese hamster ovary (CHO) cells engineered to secrete high levels of cytokine, immunological rejection of these xenogeneic cells represents a major obstacle for immunotherapeutic studies in CIA. To obviate this problem, we have attempted two different strategies. First, we have encapsulated CHO cells transfected with IL-4 or IL-13 cDNA into hollow fibers and implanted this material in the peritoneal cavity of CII-immunized DBA/1 mice. Such treatment induced a long-lasting suppressive effect on arthritis severity. Second, we aimed at permitting the prolongation of CHO survival *in vivo* by introducing the gene of Fas ligand (FasL) into the CHO/IL-4 cells. The expression of FasL on CHO/IL-4 cells potentiated the *in vivo* anti-inflammatory effect of the cytokine in CIA. However, the therapeutic effect did not result from a prolonged *in vivo* secretion of IL-4 by engineered cells since, paradoxically, FasL transfected cells underwent accelerated rejection. FasL-mediated elimination of activated neutrophils was rather suspected to participate in the down-regulation of inflammation.

Thus, the mouse model of CIA represents a very rewarding model for the investigation of new therapeutic strategies and may offer a hope of more selective interventions for the treatment of human autoimmune diseases.

Introduction

Rheumatoid arthritis (RA) is an autoimmune disease with unknown etiology that is characterized by a chronic inflammation of the synovial joints and infiltration by blood-derived cells, such as memory T cells, macrophages and plasma cells, all of which show signs of activation. These events lead in most cases to progressive destruction of cartilage and bone which is believed to result from cytokine-mediated induction of matrix metalloproteinases.

Type II collagen (CII) was identified earlier as an arthritogenic protein in rodents and primates. Thus, immunization of susceptible strains of rats [1] or mice [2] with CII in adjuvant was shown to induce a polyarthritis that mimics clinical and histological manifestations of RA. While CII obviously is not the cause of RA, it is the case that collagen immunity is a feature of the human disease and therefore, the model of collagen-induced arthritis (CIA) represents a useful tool to elaborate therapeutic approaches. In our laboratory, we have used the mouse model raised in the susceptible DBA/1 (H-2^q) strain immunized with native CII from bovine origin. The resulting disease occurs one month after antigen priming and is generally monophasic leading to spontaneous regression of clinical signs of arthritis. Interestingly, immunization with homologous CII is accompanied by a remitting perpetuated disease lasting for months [3].

The pivotal role of T cells in driving the process of mouse CIA has been widely demonstrated over the past decade allowing the development of therapeutic strategies which selectively target the autoaggressive T cells (Fig. 1). Undoubtedly, the trimolecular complex of T cell receptor (TCR), antigenic peptide and major histocompatibility complex (MHC) is the most appropriate target for specific and long-lasting therapy [4]. However, the lack of identified disease-inducing antigens in RA prompted the scientists to develop alternative approaches aimed at counteracting the proinflammatory effect of cytokines such as IL-1β or TNF-α [5]. In our laboratory, we have focused on these different therapeutic approaches that we use to immunomodulate CIA in mice.

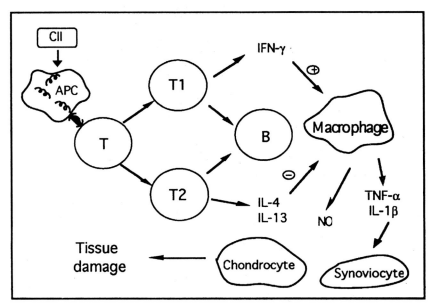

Fig. 1. Pathogenesis of murine collagen-induced arthritis.

T-Cell Targeted Immunointervention

The therapeutic use of monoclonal antibodies (mAbs) that could accurately target subsets of T cells involved in basic pathogenic mechanisms of CIA was the first approach that we concentrated on few years ago. Thus, we attempted to modulate CIA after administration of mAbs directed to eight different TCR Vβ families. We have shown that long-term elimination of T cells expressing the TCR Vβ 8.1 and TCR Vβ 8.2 prevented the development of arthritis in CII-immunized DBA/1 mice (Fig. 2) and reduced the specific humoral response. The inhibition of clinical signs in the treated mice was comparable to that achieved upon depletion of total $CD4^+$ T cells. Conversely, the administration of the other anti-TCR Vβ mAbs utilized only marginally affected the course of CIA [6]. These data point to a role for T cells expressing the TCR Vβ 8 during the induction process of CIA but do not imply that these cells are CII-specific.

To investigate the involvement of T cells reacting with CII in CIA modulation, we have generated anti-CII hybrid T cell clones. The selection of $CD4^+$ T hybridomas was performed on the basis of antigen-induced IL-2 secretion and that of $CD8^+$ hybridomas on the cytotoxic potential against CII-pulsed macrophages. Using the T cell vaccination protocol pioneered by I. Cohen [7], these clones were irradiated and injected i.v. three weeks prior to priming DBA/1 mice with CII. The different $CD4^+$ T hybridomas proved to exert opposite effects either downregulating or aggravating the disease whereas a control anti-ovalbumin T hybridoma did not alter CIA [8]. On the other hand, successful prevention against the experimental disease could be achieved with two irradiated anti-CII CD8$^+$ clones. This suppression was antigen- and disease-specific since inoculation of the clones did not affect experimental autoimmune thyroiditis. Most importantly, one of the CD8$^+$ clones had a therapeutic effect on CIA when injected after the onset of the disease [9].

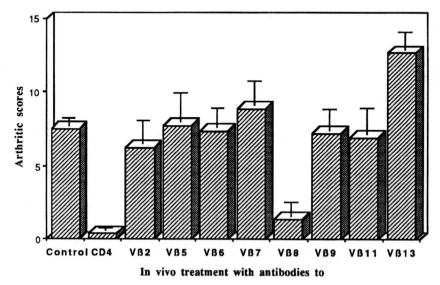

Fig. 2.   Effect of therapy with anti-TCR Vβ monoclonal antibodies on murine collagen-induced arthritis.

The mechanisms underlying the beneficial effect of T cell vaccination in experimental autoimmunity were reported to involve the generation of CD8$^+$ anti-clonotypic T cells that inhibit autoaggressive T cell subsets [10]. Evidence for the emergence of such clonotype-specific regulatory T cells in vaccinated animals was provided in the encephalomyelitis (EAE) model and moreover, it was shown that the suppressive effect can equally be achieved by immunization with TCR peptides from hypervariable regions of the pathogenic cells. Recently, similar mechanisms were suspected to be involved in the control of CIA [11].

Immune Deviation as Therapy for Autoimmune Diseases

Since the description of two antagonist subsets of CD4$^+$ T cells identified by their cytokine profile it has become increasingly apparent that the Th1-type responses are involved in the pathogenesis of certain organ-specific autoimmune disorders (Fig. 3). To study the dichotomy in the respective roles of Th1 and Th2 cells in CIA, we have established CII-specific T cell lines from lymph nodes collected at different times after immunization of DBA/1 mice with CII. Our data revealed that 60% of the lines generated eight days after priming display a mixed lymphokine secretion pattern characteristic of Th0 cells, 25% are Th1 (secreting IFN-γ) and only 15% develop a Th2 phenotype producing IL-4 and IL-5. Thereafter, during the course of the disease, the CII-specific CD4$^+$ T cell response progressively shifts to a clear Th2 phenotype which is believed to contribute to the regression of CIA [12].

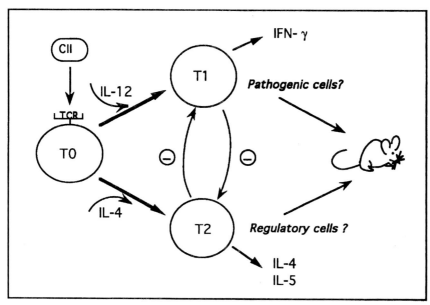

Fig. 3. Immune deviation as therapy for autoimmune diseases. It is generally accepted that upon immunization with type II collagen (CII), autoreactive T cells are stimulated and differentiate into IFN-γ producing Th1 cells that initiate the pathogenic events of collagen arthritis. Conversely, the IL-4 producing Th2 clones are postulated to exert a protective effect on the ongoing disease. Based on this hypothesis, IL-4-induced immune deviation should be a promising therapeutic approach for human diseases characterized by exaggerated Th1-like responses.

From our laboratory and from others, it appears that CD4$^+$ T cells expressing the Th1 phenotype are crucial initiators of the response in CIA. To further address this question, we have generated anti-CII Th1 clones from mice primed one week before. A T cell clone, named A 9, has been repeatedly isolated from lymph nodes of DBA/1 mice undergoing CIA. The TCR α chain of this clone expresses Vα17/Jα20 gene products and the β chain is the product of Vβ10/Dβ1.1/Jβ2.5 gene rearrangements. Interestingly, this clone shares identical α chain with two of the CII-specific T cell hybridomas used in the T cell vaccination experiments described above and, moreover, homologous CDR3 β chains associated with other Vβ families, Vβ1 and Vβ4 [8]. The fine specificity of these recurrent T cell clones is located within the arthritogenic CB11 fragment of CII. Using sequential enzymatic procedures, we could assign the recognition to a glycosylated peptide starting from residue

253 which contains a peptide a previously described as immunodominant [13] and tolerogenic [14].

Arguments indicating that clone A9 may participate in the pathogenesis of CIA come from transfer experiments. Indeed, although the clone injected alone into naive mice does not promote arthritis, when inoculated to CII-immunized mice it exacerbates the clinical signs of arthritis and enhances the anti-CII antibody response. These findings will allow to consider different protocols of peptidic or nucleotidic vaccinations to elaborate approaches for selective modulation of T cell responses.

Tipping the Th1/Th2 Cytokine Balance

Understanding of the role of cytokines during immune responses should allow to establish protocols that selectively target cytokine patterns and biological functions of cells involved in inflammatory autoimmune diseases [5]. For example, in a Th1-mediated disease, such as CIA, antagonizing IL-12 or IFN-γ should result in the downregulation of the pathogenic process. Actually, we have shown, few years ago that neutralization of endogenous IFN-γ during the initiation phase of CIA causes a profound suppression of clinical and histological signs of arthritis (Figure 4). However, if the treatment with mAb to IFN-γ is administered after onset of CIA , the effect is opposite and the articular inflammation is aggravated, thus, pointing to a biphasic effect of this cytokine during the course of arthritis [15].

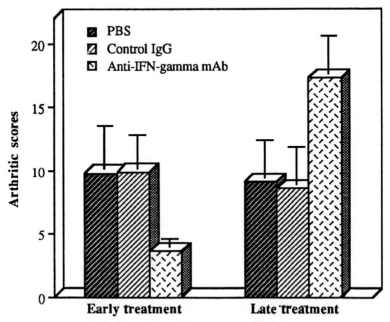

Fig. 4. Dual effect of IFN-γ during the course of collagen-induced arthritis in DBA/1 mice. Early treatment is administered during preclinical phase of the disease (D 0 to D + 28) and late treatment starts after clinical onset (D + 40 to D + 68).

The complexity of the role of IFNγ in CIA is further emphasized in our experiments using mice knockout for the IFN-γ receptor gene. In these mice, the cytokine is produced but is not functional due to the lack of specific receptors. The mice were backcrossed onto DBA/1 background to confer susceptibility to CIA and immunized with CII using the standard protocol. Unexpectedly, the mice with a disrupted gene for the IFN-γ receptor develop severe arthritis with significant earlier onset of clinical symptoms than the wild-type mice [16]. Moreover, the immunization of the mutant mice result in the generation of CII-specific T cells belonging to the Th1 phenotype that recognize the same immunodominant peptides as do DBA/1 mice.

Collectively, such intriguing data, also reported for the neutralization of IL-12 [17], will undoubtedly limit the potential use of Th1 cytokine blockers for clinical application.

The alternative approach to interfere with the Th1/Th2 balance includes the use of Th2 cytokines that exhibit the potentiality to counteract the ongoing inflammatory process through both their antagonistic action on the production of Th1 cytokines and their inhibitory effects on macrophage functions (Fig. 3). Thus, administration of IL-10 in a curative protocol was reported to ameliorate CIA [18]. In our laboratory, we have used a strategy of cellular gene therapy (via the injection of xenogeneic vector cells transfected with a plasmid construct of cytokine) to administrate IL-4 or IL-13 during the preclinical phase of CIA (Figure 5). Incidence and severity of arthritis were significantly reduced in IL-4- and IL-13- treated mice compared to control

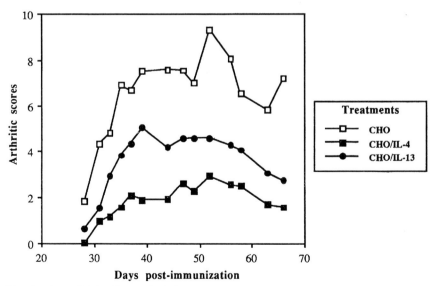

Fig. 5.   **Beneficial effects of IL-4 and IL-13 on murine collagen-induced arthritis. Cytokines were administered on days +10 and +25 post-priming via the subcutaneous engraftment of CHO cells engineered to secrete high levels of murine IL-4 (CHO/IL-4) or murine IL-13 (CHO/IL-13). Control animals received nontransfected cells (CHO).**

groups receiving nontransfected cells [19]. The beneficial effects of these Th2 cytokines seem to mainly rely on their ability to block the production of proinflammatory cytokines as evidenced by the strong decrease in TNF-α and IL-1β mRNA expression caused by inoculation of engineered cells into TNF-α transgenic mice [20].

Although the strategy of cellular gene therapy that we used proves to be powerful, the engraftment of chinese hamster ovary (CHO) fibroblasts as vector cells results in immunological rejection, thereby limiting the possibility of prolonged treatments. This problem was first circumvented by encapsulating transfected CHO cells into hollow fibers that are permeable to the cytokine secreted by the cells while protecting from xenograft rejection. After *in viro* culture of fibers filled with engineered CHO cells which allow the production of high levels of cytokines, CII-immunized DBA/1 mice were transplanted intra-peritoneally with these fibers. A long-lasting inhibition of CIA was observed in the groups of mice implanted with fibers containing CHO/IL-4 and CHO/IL-13 cells compared to the controls receiving CHO/β-galactosidase (β-gal) cells, Thus, encapsulation of secreting cells into hollow fibers seems to be an appropriate method for the long-term delivery of anti-inflammatory cytokines. Moreover, the treatment offers the advantage of possible disconti-nuation at any moment by removing the system.

The other way that we envisaged to prolong the *in vivo* survival of CHO cells was derived from the recent demonstration that successful prevention of allograft rejection can be obtained by means of cells expressing the ligand of Fas (FasL) based on their ability to deliver a signal of death to Fas$^+$ alloactivated T cells [21]. To achieve this goal, we have transfected FasL cDNA into CHO/IL-4 cells and show that these cells induce *in vitro* apoptosis of Fas$^+$ cells. We then determined whether the expression of FasL would elicit a curative effect of the cytokine on CIA by influencing the *in vivo* survival of the xenogeneic cells. DBA/1 mice were immunized with type II collagen and treated with low doses of transfected CHO cells at onset of arthritis. Severe CIA developed in the control groups injected with PBS or CHO/β-gal cells whether or not FasL cDNA was co-transfected. Likewise, engraftment of infra-therapeutic doses of CHO/IL-4 failed to alter the course of arthritis. In contrast, administration of CHO/IL-4/FasL cells markedly reduced the clinical severity and resulted in a sustained suppressive effect. However, counter to our expectation, the expression of FasL by CHO cells shortened the *in vivo* survival of the xenogeneic cells. The inoculation of CHO/IL-4/FasL cells had no influence on the proportions of lymphocyte subsets but it was associated with a decrease in circulating Mac 1$^+$ neutrophils. These findings suggest that the mechanism underlying the curative effect of IL-4 delivered by cells expressing FasL may involve the combination of the anti-inflammatory properties of IL-4 and the apoptosis of Fas$^+$ Mac1$^+$ granulocytes participating to the pathogenic process. Further investigations are required to determine whether the use of syngeneic vector cells (instead of CHO cells) cotransfected with IL-4 and FasL genes would amplify the beneficial effects of cellular gene therapy.

Concluding Remarks

Selective modulation of T-cell responses in autoimmunity has been achieved convincingly in experimental model of autoimmunity and in that regard, CIA has proven to be a suitable model to elaborate new strategies of immunotherapy. However, an obvious question is whether they may represent realistic therapies for the treatment of rheumatoid arthritis.

Undoubtedly, approaches for immune intervention aimed at targeting the TCR-peptide MHC complex involved in autoimmune responses represent powerful methods to confer highly specific long-lasting prevention of the experimental diseases. Although they are promising in theory, their extrapolation to human situation is limited by the little progress in identifying candidate disease-inducing antigens in rheumatoid arthritis. Based on the assumption that cartilage-specific antigens, such as CII, could contribute to disease perpetuation, it was attempted, few years ago, to induce oral tolerance by feeding patients with chicken CII [22]. The authors found some clinical improvement in the treated patients but these findings remain controversial.

Alternative modalities for immunomodulation of autoimmunity includes strategies interfering at a downstream step of the pathogenic events. Cytokines have already provided good targets for imunotherapy. The most successful application developed so far in rheumatoid arthritis, has been evidenced by the efficacy of an anti-TNF-α chimeric mAb [23]. Although some patients eventually relapsed, the treatment gave considerable clinical benefit and a marked decrease in inflammation. These encouraging results emphasized the critical role of TNF-α in the pathogenesis of rheumatoid arthritis and prompted the investigators to further explore the efficacy of other TNF-α antagonists (soluble TNF-α receptor p55). Likewise, neutralization of IL-1 or blockade of its receptor via the administration of the natural IL-1 receptor antagonist (IL-1ra) were shown to inhibit the inflammatory aspects in different experimental models [24]. The first trial in humans is currently in progress to evaluate the effects of inoculation into the joints of autologous synoviocytes transfected *ex vivo* with IL-1ra. Such gene therapy protocol designed to counteract local inflammation can be extended to a variety of physiologic inhibitors for metalloproteinases enzymes which are thought to be responsible for joint tissue damage.

References

1. Trentham, D.E., A.S. Townes and A.H. Kang. 1977. Autoimmunity to type II collagen: an experimental model of arthritis. *J. Exp. Med.* **146:** 857.
2. Courtenay, J.S., M.J. Dallman, A.D. Dayan, A. Martin and B. Mosedale. 1980.

Immunisation against heterologous type II collagen induces arthritis in mice. *Nature* **283**: 666.

3. Boissier, M.C., X.Z. Feng, A. Carlioz, R. Roudier and C. Fournier. 1987. Experimental autoimmune arthritis in mice. I.: Homologous type II collagen is responsible for self-perpetuating chronic polyarthritis. *Ann. Rheum. Dis.* **46**: 691.

4. Adorini, L., J.C. Guéry, G. Rodriguez-Tarduchy and S. Trembleau. 1993. Selective immunosuppression. *Immunol. Today* **14**: 285.

5. Brennan, F.M. 1994. Role of cytokines in experimental arthritis. *Clin. Exp. Immunol.* **97**: 1.

6. Chiocchia, G., M.C. Boisser and C. Fournier. 1991. Therapy against murine collagen-induced arthritis with T cell receptor Vβ-specific antibodies. *Eur. J. Immunol.* **21**: 2899.

7. Ben-Nun, A., H. Wekerle, and I. Cohen. 1981. Vaccination against autoimmune encephalomyelitis with T lymphocyte line cells reactive against myelin basic protein. *Nature* **292**: 60.

8. Chiocchia, G., B. Manoury-Schwartz, M.C. Boissier, H. Gahery, P.N. Marche, and C. Fournier. 1994. T cell regulation of collagen-induced arthritis in mice. III.: Is T cell vaccination a valuable therapy: *Eur. J. Immunol.* **24**: 2775.

9. Chiocchia, G., M.C. Boissier, B. Manoury, and C. Fournier. 1993. T cell regulation of collagen-induced arthritis in mice. II.: Immunomodulation of arthritis by cytotoxic T cell hybridomas specific for type II collagen. *Eur. J. Immunol.* **23**: 327.

10. Lider, O., T. Reshef, E. Beraud, A. Ben-Nun, and I.R. Cohen. 1988. Anti-idiotypic network induced by T cell vaccination against experimental autoimmune encephalomyelitis. *Science* **239**: 181.

11. Kumar, V., F. Aziz, E. Sercarz, and A. Miller. 1997. Regulatory T cells specific for the same framework 3 region of the Vβ8.2 chain are involved in the control of collagen-induced arthritis and experimental autoimmune encephalomyelitis. *J. Exp. Med.* **185**: 1725.

12. Doncarli, A., L.M. Stasiuk, C. Fournier, and O. Abensira-Amar. 1997. *In vivo* conversion from an early dominant Th0/Th1 response towards a Th2 phenotype during the development of collagen-induced arthritis. *Eur. J. Immunol.* **27**: 1451.

13. Brand, D.D., L.K Myers, K. Terato, K.B. Whittington, J.M. Stuart, A.H. Kang, and E.W. Rosloniec. 1994. Characterization of the T cell determinants in the induction of autoimmune arthritis by bovine α1(II)-CB11 in H-2^q mice. *J. Immunol.* **152**: 3088.

14. Khare, S.D., C.J. Krco, M.M. Griffiths, H.S. Luthra and C.S. David. 1995. Oral administration of an immunodominant human collagen peptide modulates collagen-induced arthritis. *J. Immunol.* **155**: 3653.

15. Boissier, M.C., G. Chiocchia, N. Bessis, J. Hajnal, G. Garotta, F. Nicoletti and C. Fournier. 1995. Biphasic effect of interferon-γ in murine collagen-induced arthritis. *Eur. J. Immunol.* **25**: 1184.

16. Manoury-Schwartz, B., G. Chiocchia, N. Bessis, O. Abehsira-Amar, F. Batteux, S. Muller, S. Huang, M.C. Boissier, and C. Fournier. 1997. High susceptibility to collagen-induced arthritis in mice lacking interferon-γ receptors *J. Immunol.* **158**: 5501.

17. Joosten, L.A.B., E. Lubberts, M.M.A. Helsen, and W.B. van den Berg. 1997. Dual role of IL-12 in early and late stages of murine collagen type II arthritis. *J. Immunol.* **159**: 4094.

18. Walmsley, M., P.D. Katsikis, E. Abney, S. Parry, R.O. Williams, R.N. Maini, and M. Feldmann. 1996. Interleukin-10 inhibition of the progression of established collagen-induced arthritis. *Arthritis Rheum.* **39**: 495.

19. Bessis, N., M.C. Boissier, P. Ferrara, T. Blankenstein, D. Fradelizi and C. Fournier. 1996. Attenuation of murine collagen-induced arthritis by treatment with vector cells engineered to secrete interleukin-13. *Eur. J. Immunol.* **26:** 2399.

20. Bessis, N., G. Chiocchia, G. Kollias, A. Minty, C. Fournier, D. Fradelizi, and M.C. Boissier. 1998. Modulation of proinflammatory cytokine production in tumor necrosis factor-alpha (TNF-α)-transgenic mice by treatment with cells engineered to secrete IL-4, IL-10 or IL-13. *Clin. Exp. Immunol.* **111:** 391.

21. Lau, H.T., M.Yu., A. Fontana, C.J. Stoeckert Jr. 1996. Prevention of islet allograft rejection with engineered myoblasts expressing FasL in mice. *Science (Wash. DC)* **273:** 109.

22. Trentham, D.E., R.A. Dynesius-Trentham, E.J. Orav, D. Combitchi, C. Lorenzo, K.L. Sewel, D.A. Hafler and H.L. Weiner. 1993. Effects of oral administration of type II collagen on rheumatoid arthritis. *Science* **261:** 1727.

23. Eliott, M.J., R.N. Maini, M. Feldmann, A. Long-Fox, P. Charles, P. Katsikis, F.M. Brennan, J. Walker, H. Bijl, J. Ghrayeb and J.N. Woody. 1993. Treatment of rheumatoid arthritis with chimeric monoclonal antibodies to tumor necrosis factor α. *Arthritis Rheum.* **36:** 1681.

24. Bandara, G., G.M. Mueller, J. Galea-Lauri, M.H. Tindal, H.I. Georgescu, M.K. Suchanek, G.L. Hung, J.C. Glorioso, P.D. Robbins and C.H. Evans. 1993. Intraarticular expression of biologically active IL-1 receptor antagonist protein by *ex vivo* gene transfer. *Proc. Natl. Acad. Sci. (USA)* **90:** 10764.

Immunopharmacology: Strategies for immunotherapy
S.N. Upadhyay (Ed)

14. Immunomodulatory Effect of Slow Acting Anti-Rheumatic Drugs (SAARDs)

S. Naik, R. Yadav, A. Mangalam and R. Misra
Department of Immunology, Sanjay Gandhi Postgraduate Institute of
Medical Sciences, Lucknow-226014, India

Introduction

Rheumatoid arthritis (RA) is a slowly progressing chronic autoimmune disorder. The major pathology is in the joint where a progressive destruction of joint tissue results in multiple deformities and severe morbidity. Although the exact etiological agent is unknown, it is believed than an arthritogenic peptide gains access to the joint and generates an immune response, which is directed against synovial tissue. During disease progression monocytes and macrophages infiltrate the synovium and secrete large quantities of proinflammatory cytokines mainly Interleukine-1 (IL-1), Tumor necrosis factor α (TNα) and Interleukine-6 (IL-6) (Burmester $et\ al$ 1983), which appear to play a central role in disease pathogenesis (Buchan $et\ al.$ 1988, Alvaro-Gracia $et\ al$ 1989). Increased level of IL-1, TNFα, IL-6, Interleukine-8 (IL-8) and Interferon γ (IFNγ) in synovial fluid along with increased amount of mRNA have been demonstrated in cells infiltrating the synovium of RA patients. TNFα appears to play a critical role in mediating synovitis as a chimeric anti-TNFα antibody has been shown to give marked clinical benefit (Elliott $et\ al$ 1994). Down regulation of TNFα was found to secondarily decrease IL-1 and IL-6 levels (Fong $et\ al,$ 1989).

Treatment of RA include drugs to control inflammation e.g. nonsteroidal anti-inflammatory drugs (NSAIDs) and slow acting anti-inflammatory drugs (SAARDs) which probably induce regression or arrest progression of the disease. Drugs in this group include gold compounds (e.g. Gold Sodium thiomalate (GSTM), auranofin), D-pencillamine (D-pen), chloroquine, methotrexate (MTX) and sulfasalazine. These drugs also have tissue protective effect. Exact mechanism of action of these drugs in RA is not very well understood but it is thought that SAARDs can exert their beneficial role by influencing cytokine network and immune reactivity.

The limitation of SAARD therapy, however, is their well-known toxicity and the variation in clinical efficacy (Furst, 1985). This results in 30–40% of patients having to change from one drug to another. Hence, there has been an interest in finding markers for predicting toxicity as well as clinical response. Heterogeneity among normal individual and RA patients in their ability to synthesize pro-inflammatory cytokines spontaneously and on LPS activation has been reported. This along with the observed variations in the ability of GSTM to inhibit *in vitro* IL-1β production (Danis *et al,* 1990), raises the possibility that this may be related to the *in vitro* response to drug.

There have been a number of studies reporting the effect of SAARDs on proinflammatory cytokines. Auranofin has been shown to inhibit *in vitro* IFNγ production by Con-A stimulated PBMCs of RA patients and normal controls (Harth *et al.* 1990). Sequential synovial biopsies in-patients on chrysotherapy have shown decreased m RNA levels of IL-1α, IL-1β, IL-6 and TNFα (Yanni *et al,* 1994). GSTM has also been shown to bind to SH groups of protein kinase C (PKC) and inhibit AP-1, AP-2 TF-IId and NF-IL6 (Handell *et al,* 1993), which are transcription factor for the pro-inflammatory cytokines. Following MTX therapy, spontaneous production of IL-1β and TNFα was significantly decreased (Olsen *et al.* 1987 and Barrera *et al.* 1994). There is no report on the action of D-pen on proinflammatory cytokines. The present study was therefore undertaken to evaluate *in vitro* effect of GSTM, MTX and D-pen on spontaneous and LPS stimulated proinflammatory cytokine production by the peripheral blood mononuclear cells of patients with RA. An attempt was also made to asses whether *in vitro* response can be used to predict *in vivo* response.

Patients and Methods

Fortytwo patients with active RA who fulfilled modified ACR criteria (Arnett *et al.* 1990) were included in the study. None of them had received SAARD or steroids before their entry into the study. Patients were started on monotherapy with either GSTM (*n* = 16) or MTX (*n* = 26), after assessment of disease activity and venous blood sampling for *in vitro* studies. All the patients were evaluated for disease activity parameters (early morning stiffness, number of swollen joints, Ritchie articular index, visual analog scale) at the beginning of study and after 6 months of the therapy. Study was conducted in two phases—thirty in first phase (15 each in GSTM and MTX group) and twelve in the second phase (1 in GSTM and 11 in MTX group).

PBMC Isolation and culture

All reagents used for isolation of peripheral blood mononuclear cells (PBMC) were endotoxin free. PBMCs were separated from venous blood by density gradient sedimentation on lymphoprep. Following three washings with phosphate buffered saline (PBS), 0.15M pH7.2, the cells were suspended in RPMI-1640, supplemented with 10% fetal calf serum, 0.1% antibiotic mixture, L. glutamine and HEPES (CRPMI) and adjusted to a concentration of 1×10^6 cells/ml. One ml cultures were set up in round bottom culture tubes with varying doses of either GSTM, MTX or D-pen in the presence and absence of 10ng per ml of LPS. Cultures were incubated for 24 hrs at 37°C in 95% humidity and 5% CO_2 atmosphere. The tubes were centrifuged and the culture supernatants containing secreted cytokines were harvested and stored at –70°C.

TNF-α Bioassay

L-929, a murine fibroblast cell line (NCCS, Pune, India) was grown in 25 cm^2-culture flask to log phase. The cells were trypsinized and washed thrice in RPMI 1640 and resuspended in CRPMI at a concentration of 2×10^5 cells/ml in presence of Actinomycin D. 100 μl of cell suspension was added to each well of 96 well flat bottom microtiter plate and incubated at 37°C, in 5% CO_2, 95% air for 24 hrs. 100 μl of 1:10 dilution of culture supernatant or different dilution of recombinant TNFα were added to wells in duplicate. Plate was incubated at 37°C in 5% CO_2, 95% air for 24 hrs. 10 μl of 5 mg/ml MTT in RPMI was added to each well and this was followed 4 hrs later by addition of 100 µl of lysis buffer. The plate was read at 540 nm in an ELISA reader. Specificity of the cell line was confirmed by failure to induce cytotoxicity of L-929 by TNFα in the presence of neutralizing polyclonal anti-TNFα antibody. The inter assay variation was 10% and intra assay precision was 15%.

IL-6 Bioassay

The IL 6 bioassay was performed as described by Aarden *et al* (1987). An IL-6 dependent human B cell line B9 (Dr. L. Aarden, Netherlands) was grown in 25 cm^2 flask up to log phase. The cell were then washed thrice with plain RPMI and the cell suspension was added to 96 well flat bottom culture plate. 100 μl of various dilutions of culture supernatants were added in duplicate along with the recombinant IL-6. The plate was incubated at 37°C in 5% CO_2, 95% air for 72 hrs and cell viability was assessed using MTT as described for TNF-α. Results were calibrated against those of the recombinant standards. Specificity of cell line was confirmed by the failure to induce proliferation of the cells by IL-6 in the presence of appropriate polyclonal antibody. The inter assay variation was 18% and intra assay variation was 16%.

IL-1β Bioassay

The IL-1β assay was performed as described by Morinaga *et al.* [1990]. A human keratanocyte cell line A-375 (NCCS, Pune, India) cells was grown in 25 cm^2 culture flask to log phase. The cell were typsinized and washed thrice with plain RPMI and suspended in CRPMI at a cell concentration of 1×10^5 cell per ml. 50 μl of the cell suspension and 50 μl of culture supernatant or dilution of the recombinant IL-1β were added to wells in duplicate. The plate was incubated at 37°C in 5% CO_2, 95% air for 72 hrs and cell viability was assessed using MTT as described for TNFα. Results were calibrated against those of the recombinant standards. Specificity of cell line was confirmed by the failure to inhibit proliferation by IL-1β in the presence of appropriate polyclonal antibody The inter assay variation was 15% and intra assay variation was 13%.

In vitro Response

Reduction in cytokine production in presence of SAARD when compared to the cytokine production in absence of SAARD was defined as *in vitro* response. Percentage inhibition was calculated as:

$$\% \text{ inhibition} = \frac{\text{Cytokine levels with LPS} - \text{Cytokine levels with LPS} + \text{Drug}}{\text{Cytokine levels with LPS}} \times 100$$

Statistical Analysis

Paired data were analyzed using the nonparametric Wilcoxon Rank sum test. The results are expressed as median + range.

In vivo-in vitro correlation was analyzed by chi-square test.

Results

Clinical Response to GSTM and MTX

Fifteen patients each were started on monotherapy with GSTM and MTX. The mean disease activity score for each group at the start of therapy and at the end of 6 months of therapy is given in Table 1.

Table 1. **Response of disease activity parameters to SAARD therapy (mean ± SD)**

Drug	Parameter	0 month	6 months
GSTM (n = 15)	Early morning stiffness[a]	111 ± 65	50 ± 42
	No of swollen joints	6 ± 3	4 ± 3
	Ritchie articular index[b]	14 ± 5	8 ± 5
	Visual analog scole[c]	5 ± 1	3 ± 2
MTX (n = 15)	Early morning stiffness[a]	119 ± 64	58 ± 42
	No of swollen joints	6 ± 3	4 ± 3
	Ritchie articular index[b]	19 ± 6	14 ± 10
	Visual analog scale[c]	4 ± 1	3 ± 2

[a] In minutes
[b] Number of painful joints
[c] On a score of 0–10

Effect of GSTM on LPS Stimulated Cytokine Production

The median LPS induced TNFα production by PBMC from patients with RA (70 IU/ml; range 21-900 IU/ml) was significantly higher (P < 0.02) than the spontaneous TNFα production median (40 IU/ml; range 8–280 IU/ml). GSTM showed significant inhibition of LPS induced TNFα production at all the doses tested. These results were confirmed in the second phase of the study in 12 patients (Table 2, Fig. 1).

Table 2.   Effect of GSTM on LPS stimulated TNFα^a (IU/ml) ($n = 30$)

Dose of GSTM (conc./ml)	Phase I ($N = 30$)	Phase II ($N = 12$)
NIL	70 (21–900)	56 (1–700)
10 μg	11* (9–420)	6* (1–600)
1 μg	15* (12–520)	10* (1–450)
100 ng	58* (1–840)	ND
10 ng	40* (1–840)	ND

*Values of TNF α in the presence of GSTM v/s absence of GSTM (P < 0.05)
[a]Values represented as a median (range)
ND—Not done

The LPS induced IL-1β production by PBMC from patients with RA (median 335 IU/ml; range 100–600 IU/ml) was significantly higher (P < 0.02) than the spontaneous IL-1β production (median 160 IU/ml; range 45–450 IU/ml). GSTM showed significant inhibition of LPS stimulated IL-1β production at 10 μg and 1 μg dose (Table 3, Fig. 1).

The LPS induced IL-6 production (median 1200 IU/mL; range 180–5000 IU/ml) was significantly higher (P < 0.02) than the spontaneous IL-6 production (median 440 IU/ml; range 100–600 IU/ml). GSTM inhibited LPS stimulated IL-6 production at all the doses tested (Table 3, Fig. 1).

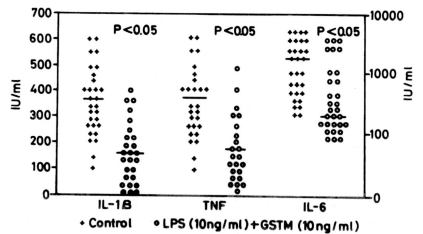

Fig. 1.   Effect of GSTM on LPS stimulated cytokine production (horizontal bar shows median value).

Table 3. Effect of GSTM on LPS stimulated IL-1β (IU/ml) and IL-6 (IU/ml)[a] (n=30)

Dose of GSTM (conc./ml)	IL-1β	IL-6
NIL	335 (100–600)	1200 (180–5000)
10 µg	65* (45–400)	420* (100–4800)
1 µg	150* (30–415)	440* (110–4000)
100 ng	215 (10–514)	180* (100–3000)
10 ng	160 (5–600)	200* (112–3600)

[a] Values represented as median (range)
*Values of IL -1β and IL-6 in the presence of GSTM v/s absence of GSTM (P < 0.05)

Effect of MTX on LPS Stimulated Cytokine Production

MTX showed significant inhibition of LPS stimulated TNFα production at 100 ng and 10 ng. These results were confirmed in subsequent groups of patients studied (Table 4, Fig. 2). MTX inhibited LPS stimulated IL-1β and IL-6 production (Table 5, Fig. 2).

Table 4. Effect of MTX on LPS stimulated TNFα[a] (IU/ml)

Dose of MTX (conc./ml)	Phase I (n = 30)	Phase II (n = 12)
NIL	70 (21–900)	58 (1–700)
100 ng	40* (8–700)	10* (1–220)
10 ng	26* (8–1000)	4.4* (1–750)

[a] Values represented as median (range)
*Values of TNFα in the presence of GSTM v/s absence of MTX (P < 0.05)

Effect of D-Pen on LPS Stimulated Cytokine Production

D-pen had no effect on overall spontaneous production of IL-1β and IL-6, at any of the doses tested; it inhibited spontaneous TNFα production at 10 µg/ml (data not shown). D-pen inhibited LPS stimulated IL-1β, TNFα all IL-6 production at all the doses tested (Table 6, Fig. 3).

Correlation of *in vivo* Response to SAARDs with *in vitro* of SAARDs

Patients with decrease of 20% or more in number of swollen joints and

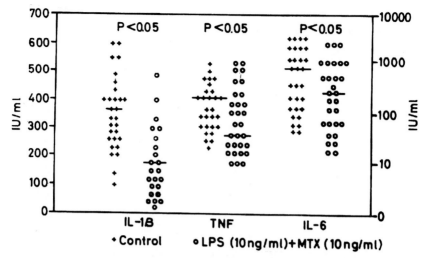

Fig. 2. Effect of MTX on LPS stimulated cytokine production (horizontal bar shows median value).

Ritchie articular index as assessed at the end of six months of therapy were labelled as *in vivo* responders. Individuals in whom the drug inhibited cytokine production by 20% or more were labeled as *in vitro* responders. Twelve of the patients each on GSTM and MTX were available for evaluation at 6 months.

Table 5. Effect of MTX on LPS stimulated IL-1β (IU/ml) and IL-6 (IU/ml)[a] (n = 30)

Dose of MTX (conc./ml)	IL-1β	IL-6
NIL	335 (100–600)	1200 (180–5000)
100 ng	240* (65–600)	360* (100–3200)
10 ng	150* (31–585)	200* (120–4800)

[a]Values represented as median (range)
*Values of IL-1β, IL-6 in the presence of MTX v/s absence of MTX ($P < 0.05$).

Response to GSTM (Table 7A, Fig. 4)

Eight of the 15 patients who were on GSTM treatment were labeled as *in vivo* responders; of these 5 showed *in vitro* response to IL-1β and remaining three were *in vitro* non-responders. Out of the 4 patients who showed *in vivo* non-response to GSTM, 2 patients were *in vitro* nonresponders to IL-1β and 2 *in vitro* responders. Therefore, the *in vitro* and *in vivo* response for GSTM and IL-1β was concordant (as response or non-response) in 7 of 12 (58%) while it was disconcordant in 5 of 12 (42%).

Of the eight patients on GSTM who were responders, 7 were *in vitro* responders to TNFα and IL-6. Out of the four patients who showed *in vivo*

Table 6. Effect of D-Pen on LPS stimulated IL-1β (IU/ml), TNFα (IU ml) and IL-6 (IU/ml)[a] (n = 30)

Dose of D-Pen (conc./ml)	IL-1β	TNFα	IL-6
NIL	335 (100–600)	70 (21–900)	1200 (180–5000)
10 μg	35* (15–395)	50* (5–1300)	420* (100–4000)
1 μg	45* (8–350)	22* (1-1100)	420* (120–4200)
100 ng	55* (19–315)	22* (7–420)	280* (80–3600)
10 ng	65* (10–500)	20* (8–220)	220* (100–2600)

[a]Values represented as median (range)
*Values of IL-1β, TNFα and IL-6 in the presence of D-pen v/s absence of D-pen (P < 0.05).

non-response to GSTM, three were *in vitro* non-responders to TNFα and IL-6. Therefore, the *in vitro* and *in vivo* response for GSTM and TNFα and GSTM and IL-6 was concordant (as response or non-response) in 10 of 12 (83%) while it was disconcordant in 2 of 12 (17%).

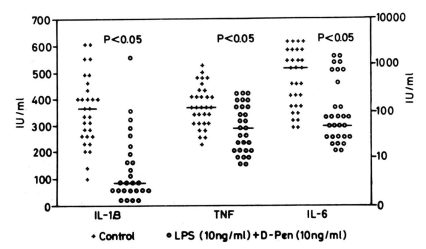

Fig. 3.   Effect of D-pen on LPS stimulated cytokine production (horizontal bar shows median value).

Response to MTX (Table 7B and Fig. 5)

Nine of the 15 patients who were on MTX treatment were *in vivo* responders and 4 patients were non-responders. Of the nine *in vivo* responders, seven were *in vitro* responders to IL-1β and the remaining two were *in vitro* non-responders. Out of the three patients who showed *in vivo* non-response, one

Table 7. *In vivo-in vitro* **correlation**

For A: GSTM

	A⁺/B⁺	A⁺/B⁻	A⁻/B⁺	A⁻/B⁻
IL-1β	5	3	2	2
TNFα	7	1	1	3
IL-6	7	1	1	3

For B: MTX

IL-1β	7	2	3	1
TNFα	5	4	2	2
IL-6	4	5	2	2

A: *in vivo*,   +: response
B: *in vitro*,   −: no response

patient was *in vitro* non-responder to IL-1β, while the remaining two patients were *in vitro* responder. Therefore, the *in vitro* and *in vivo* response to MTX and IL-1β was concordant (as response or non-response) in 8 of 13 (61%) while it was disconcordant in 5 of 13 (39%).

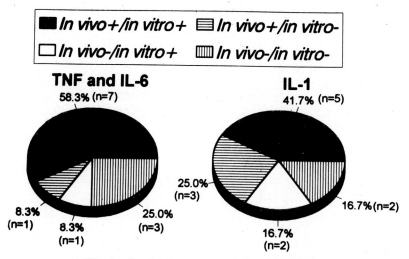

Fig. 4. In vivo-in viro correlation for GSTM.

Of nine *in vivo* responders to MTX, four were *in vitro* responders to IL-6 and five *in vitro* non-responders. Four patients who showed *in vivo* non-response to MTX, two were *in vitro* non-responders, while the remaining two patients were *in vitro* responders. Therefore, the *in vitro* and *in vivo* response for MTX and IL-6 was concordant (as response or non-response) in 6 of 13 (47%) while it was disconcordant in 7 of 13 (54%).

Of nine responders who showed *in vivo* response to MTX, 5 were *in vitro* responders to TNFα while four were *in vitro* non-responders. Of the four patients who showed *in vivo* non-response two were *in vitro* non-responders while the remaining two patients were *in vitro* responders. Therefore, the *in vitro* and *in vivo* response to MTX and TNFα was concordant (as response or non-response) in 7 of 13 (51%) while it was disconcordant in 6 of 13 (49%).

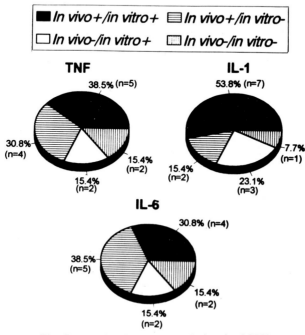

Fig. 5. *In vivo-in vitro* correlation for MTX.

The *in vitro* and *in vivo* correlation did not reach statistical significance for any of drug-cytokine combinations.

Discussion

In the present study we have made a comprehensive evaluation of the *in vitro* effect of SAARDs on proinflammatory cytokines. GSTM, MTX and D-pen failed to inhibit spontaneous IL-1β, TNFα and IL-6 production, except for D-pen, which showed inhibition of TNFα at a dose of 10 μg/ml. However these drugs inhibited LPS stimulated cytokine production from doses ranging from 10 μg/ml to 10 ng/ml except for GSTM which inhibited IL-1β only at 10 μg/ml and 1 μg/ml.

It should be pointed out that the drugs have been used in wide dosage spectrun that closely correlates with serum levels achieved during therapy. Serum gold levels in RA treated with GSTM were reported as 2–5 μg/ml (Jessop and Johns, 1973).

The possibility that inhibition found by us in the *in vitro* studies could be by direct killing of the target cells in the bioassays by residual drugs in the culture supernatant was excluded. When the drugs were tested directly on the targets, only MTX was found to have direct cytotoxic effect for B9 and A-375 cell lines (used for IL-6 and IL-1β bioassay) at the higher doses of 10 μg/ml and 1 μg/ml.

GSTM and MTX have previously been shown to cause marked inhibition of thymocyte proliferation response to IL-1β, while D-pen failed to do so. All three drugs inhibited zymosan stimulated IL-1β production (Chang et al, 1990). GSTM, at 10 μg/ml and 1 μg/ml dose has been shown to inhibit LPS stimulated in vitro IL-1β production by normal PBMCs (Danis et al. 1989; Danis et al, 1990). However, at 100 ng/ml and 10 ng/ml concentrations GSTM showed augmentation of LPS stimulated IL-1β production. We too have earlier reported that 10 μg/ml dose of GSTM augmented spontaneous TNFα production by normal PBMCs while it had no effect on spontaneous TNFα production by PBMC of patients with RA (Yadav et al, 1997). No explanation has been offered for this bimodal effect. MTX had no effect on in vitro IL-1β production although IL-1 bioactivity was inhibited (Segal et al, 1989). There are no reports on the in vitro action of D-pen on cytokine production.

Other workers have assessed the effect of SAARDs therapy on pro-inflammatory cytokines. Treatment with parenteral gold salts for 2 weeks had no effect on the cytokine response within the synovial tissues as assessed by immunohistochemical studies (Yanni et al, 1994). They found a reduction in IL-1α, IL-1β and IL-6 expression of the synovial lining cells after 12 weeks of therapy. Treatment with Auranofin but not gold sodium thiomalate was found to decrease the spontaneous IL 6 production by the PBMCs after 12 weeks of therapy, but not after 24 weeks; there was no effect on LPS-stimulated IL-6 production after 12 or 24 weeks of treatment (Crilly et al, 1994). MTX therapy of short duration has also been shown to inhibit IL-1 and IL-6 production which was not as significant as following chronic treatment (Barrera et al, 1994; Chang et al, 1992).

Our observation that SAARDs inhibit only LPS activated cytokine production in vitro and not spontaneous production suggest that these agents may act at some of the points in intracellular signaling activated by LPS and required for proinflammatory cytokine synthesis. LPS activates monocytes through cells surface CD14 leading to transcriptional activation of cytokine genes via the ceramide pathway. Ceramide activates specific PKCs, and mitogen activated protein (MAP) kinases, which in turn activate various nuclear factors responsible for initiating IL-1, TNF α and IL-6 gene transcription and cytokine production. Proinflammatory cytokines are controlled by a common set of transcription factors, which include AP-1, NF-IL-6. GSTM and D-pen are both known to bind to sulphydryl groups which are also present in the kinases and alter the functional capabilities of proteins (Mckeown et al, 1994). It is well known that gold inhibits transcriptional factors in vitro (Hashimoto et al, 1992; Handell et al, 1993). It is therefore possible to speculate that GSTM and

D-pen would exert their inhibitory effects by influencing ceramide activated PKCs which in turn would affect cytokine production.

In this study we have made the first attempt to use the *in vitro* inhibition of LPS stimulated pro-inflammatory cytokine as a predictor for *in vivo* therapeutic response. The number of patients on each drug, who continued on follow-up, was small and no statistically significant association could be found. However, the fairly high concordance rate of 83% between *in vivo* and *in vitro* response for GSTM with TNFα and IL-6 is encouraging. Studies on larger group of patients are required to give a final answer.

The drugs used in this study differ widely in their structure and although they provide relief from symptoms, their ability to retard the progression of joint destruction is limited (Pincus, 1988). Recent evidences indicate that major mediators of bone and cartilage resorption are TNFα, IL-1 and IL-6 (Odeh, 1997). The efficacy of these drugs in RA, therefore, may be a result of their action on cytokine production.

Rheumatoid arthritis is a chronic progressive disease and is responsible for a significant amount of morbidity in all populations. An effort to design more efficacious and less toxic drugs as well as improve existing drug regimes is a major international goal. Our results should help to better understand the mode of action of SAARDs and evolve better strategies for their rational use.

Acknowledgments

The authors acknowledge the kind supply of Gold Sodium Thiomalate from Dagenham Pharmaceuticals, U.K. The study was supported by a grant from the center of Scientific and Industrial Research, Government of India. The grant in aid for purchase of equipment by Japan International Co-operation Agency is also gratefully acknowledged.

References

Alvaro-Gracia J.M., Zvaifler N.J., Firestein G.S. Cytokines in chronic inflammatory arthritis. IV. GM-CSF mediated induction of class II MHC antigen on human monocytes: a possible role in RA. *J. Exp. Med.* 1989; **1146:** 865–75.

Aarden L.A., de Groot E.R., Schaap O.L., Lansdrop P.M. Production of hybridoma growth factor by human monocytes. *Eur. J. Immunol.* 1987; **17:** 1411–16.

Arnett F.C., Edworthy S.M., Bloch D.A. The American Rheumatism Association 1987 revised criteria for the classification of rheumatoid arthritis. *Arthritis Rheum* 1990; **31:** 315–324.

Barrera P. Boerbooms A.M., Demacker P.N., van de Putte L.B., Gallati H, van der Meer J.W., Circulating concentration and production of cytokines and soluble receptors in rheumatoid arthritis patients: effect of a single dose methotrexate. *Br. J. Rheumatol* 1994; **33:** 1017–24.

Buchan G., Barret K., Turner M., Chantry D., Maini R.N., Fieldman M. Interleukin-1 and tumor nerosis factor α m-RNA expression in rheumatoid arthritis: prolonged production of IL-1. *Clin. Exp. Immunol.* 1988; **73:** 449–55.

Burmester G.R., Lorcher P. Koch B., Winchester R.J., Dimitriu-Bona A., Kalden J.R., Mohr W. The tissue architecture of synovial membranes in inflammatory and non-inflammatory joint diseases. I. The localization of the major synovial cell population as detected by monoclonal reagents directed towards Ia and monocyte-macrophage antigens. *Rheumatology Int.* 1983; **3**: 173–81.

Chang D.M., Baptiste P. Schur P.H. The effect of antirheumatic drugs on Interleukin-1 (IL-1) activity and IL-1 inhibitor production by human monocytes. *J Rheumatol* 1990; **17**: 1148–57.

Chang D.M., Weinblatt M.E., Schur P.H. The effect of methtrexate on Interleukin-1 in patients with rheumatoid arthritis. *J. Rheumatol* 1992; **19**: 1678–82.

Crilly A., Madhok R., Watson J., Capell H.A., Sturrock R.D. Production of Interleukin-6 by monocytes isolated from rheumatoid arthritis patients receiving second line drug therapy. *Br. J. Rheumatol* 1994; **33**: 821–25.

Danis V.A., Kulesz A.J., Nelson D.S., Brooks P.M. Bimodal effect of Gold on Interleukin-1 production by blood monocytes (Letter). *J Rheumatol* 1989; **16**: 1160–61.

Danis V.A., Kulesz A.J., Nelson D.S., Brooks P.M. The effect of gold sodium thiomalate and auranofin on lipopolysaccharide induced Interleukin-1 production by blood monocytes *in vitro;* variation in healthy subjects and patients with arthritis. *Clin. Exp. Rheumatol* 1990; **79**: 335–40.

Elliott M.J., Maini R.N., Feldmann M., Kalden J.R., Antoni C., Smolen J.S., Leeb B., Breedveld F.C., Macfarlane J.D., Bijl H., Woody J.N. Randomised double blind comparison of a chimeric monoclonal antibody to tumor necrosis factor α (cA2) versus placebo in rheumatoid arthritis. *Lancet* 1994; **334**: 1105–10.

Fong Y., Tracey K.J., Moldawer L.L., Hesse D.G., Manogue K.B., Kenney J.S., Lee A.T., Kuo G.C., Antibodies to cachetin/tumor necrosis factor α reduce Interleukin-1 beta and Interleukin-6 during lethal bacteremia *J.Exp. Med.* 1989; **170**: 1627–33.

Furst D.E. Clinical pharmacology of very low dose methotrexate for use in rheumatoid arthritis. *J. Rheumatol.* 1985; **12**: 11–14.

Handell M.L., de Fazio A., Watts C.K., Day R.O., Sutherland R.L. Inhibition of DNA binding and transcriptional activity of a nuclear receptor transcription factor by aurothiomalate and other metal ions. *Mol. Pharmacol.* 1993; **40**: 613–18.

Harth M., Cousin K. McCain G.A. *In vitro* effects of two Gold compounds, and D-pencillamine on the production of interferon gamma. *Immunopharmacol. Immunotoxicol.* 1990; **12**: 39–60.

Hashimoto K., Whitehurst C.E., Matsubara T., Hirohata K., Lipsky P. Immunomodulatory effects of therapeutic gold compound. *J. Clin. Inv.* 1992; **89**: 1839–48.

Jessop J.D., Johns R.G. Serum gold determination in patients with rheumatoid arthritis receiving sodium aurothiomalate. *Ann. Rheum. Dis.* 1973; **32**: 228–32.

McKeown M.J., Hall N.D., Corvalan J.R. Deffective monocyte accessory function due to surface sulphydryl (-SH) oxidation in rheumatoid arthritis. *Clin. Exp. Rheumatol.* 1984; **56**: 607–13.

Morinaga Y., Hayashi H., Takeuchi A., Onozaki K. Antiproliferative effect of interleukin 1 (IL-1) on tumor cells: G0-G1 arrest of a human melanoma cell line by IL-1. *Biochem. Biophy. Res. Commun* 1990; **173**: 186–92.

Odeh M. New insight in to the pathogenesis and treatment of rheumatoid arthritis. *Clin. Immunol. Immunopathol.* 1997; **83**: 103–116.

Olsen N.J., Callahan L.F., Pincus T. Immunologic studies of rheumatoid arthritis patients treated with methotrexate. *Arthritis Rheum.* 1987; **30**: 481–88.

Pincus T. Rheumatoid arthritis: disappointing long-term outcome despite short-term clinical trials. *J. Clin. Epidemiol* 1988; **41**: 1037–41.

Segal R., Mozes E., Yaron N., Tartakovsky B. The effect of methotrexate on production and activity of Interleukin-1. *Arthritis. Rheum.* 1989; **32**: 370–77.

Yadav R., Misra R.N., Naik S. *In viro* effect of gold sodium thiomalate and methotrexate on tumor necrosis factor production in normal healthy individual and patients with rheumatoid arthritis. *Int. J. Immunopharmacol.* 1997; **19:** 111–14.

Yanni G., Nabil M., Farahat M.R., Poston R.N., Panayi G.S. Intramuscular gold decreases cytokine expression and macrophage numbers in the synovial membrane. *Ann. Rheum. Dis.* 1994; **53:** 315–22.

Immunopharmacology: Strategies for immunotherapy
S.N. Upadhyay (Ed)
Copyright © 1999 Narosa Publishing House, New Delhi, India

15. Modulation of Nitric Oxide (NO) Production of Macrophages by Plant Derived Immunomodulators as Therapeutic Strategy Against Tumors and Intracellular Infections

Shakti N. Upadhyay
National Institute of Immunology, New Delhi, India

Disease manifestation is basically a result of either inadequate or uncontrolled immune response of the host against a pathogen. While immunodeficiency may facilitate infections, an uncontrolled or exaggerated immune response against a pathogen may also be deleterious or undesirable for the host. Immunocompetence of the host therefore depends on a controlled or balanced immune response to a potential pathogenic stimulus.

Macrophages are central to host defense and they not only form the first line of defense against pathogens and but also help in the generation of specific and long term immunity. Macrophages are thus involved in both the afferent and efferent arms of the immune system—former in antigen processing and presentation and latter as a major effector cells that contain and kill intracellular pathogens. One of the current opinions in immunology is that "a mammalian host unable to activate its macrophages to a state of heightened microbial resistance is susceptible to infection by an intracellular pathogen" (Nathan and Hibbs, 1991). Although phagolysosomal products of macrophages are sufficient to neutralize, degrade and eliminate most foreign bodies, certain infectious pathogens resist this first line of defense and actually thrive within the macrophages, possibly by down-regulating the anti-microbial defense mechanisms of macrophages. It appears that during the evolutionary course of host-parasite interactions, many parasites have acquired the ability to survive within the host by parasitizing and affecting the immunocompetence of the macrophages. The role of macrophage is therefore crucial for an effective protection against tumor and infections.

Recent studies have shown that in addition to reactive oxygen intermediates (ROIs) such as free oxygen radicals, macrophages also produce reactive nitrogen intermediates (RNIs), i.e., nitric oxide (NO), as effector molecules, NO, a labile and highly reactive gas, which acts as cytotoxic/cytostatic effector molecule against tumor cells (Hibbs et al., 1987 a, b) and various intracellular and extracellular pathogens (James, 1995). Many of the tumors and intracellular pathogens survive by down-regulating the ability of macrophages to produce NO. One of the possible therapeutic strategies against tumors and infections, therefore, could be to upregulate or restore production of NO in tumor-bearing or parasitized hosts.

Regulation of NO production

NO production in activated macrophages results from enzymatic oxidative deimination and conversion of L-arginine to L-citrulline. In the process, NO is generated from one of the guanidino nitrogens; NO then undergoes oxidative degradation to form nitrite (NO_2) and nitrate (NO_3) (Moncada and Higgs, 1995; Knowles and Moncada, 1994). Three different forms of Nitric Oxide Synthase (NOS) representing three different gene products, have been identified in different cell types (Marletta, 1994). In contrast to the constitutive form of NOS (cNOS) present in endothelial cells and neurons, macophage NOS is inducible (iNOS) and is expressed in response to certain cytokines or bacterial LPS. It has now been shown that murine mactrophages must receive two consecutive signals in order to produce NO. While IFN-γ is the most common primary signal for macrophage activation, TNF-α produced by the macrophages in response to bacterial LPS or any parasite provides the second signal as an autocrine stimulus (Drapier et al. 1988). Recent studies have shown that conversion of L-arginine within macrophages may follow two different enzymatic pathways depending on the cytokines. While cytokines of Th-1 type (IFN-γ, IL-2, TNF-α) activate NOS pathway and enhance conversion of L-arginine into citrulline and NO production, cytokines of Th-2 type (IL-4, IL-10, TGF-β) activate arginase which coverts L-arginine into ornithine and urea and consequently NO production is down regulated (Modolell *et al.*, 1995).

The ability of human monocytes to produce NO has been a subject of much debate. However, it is being realized that most of studies carried out with human monocytes were on the freshly isolated cells from peripheral blood, which may not be physiologically competent to produce NO. Recent studies suggest that the signals required for human monocytes to produce NO may be different from those of murine macrophages. In fact, crosslinking of CD-69, an integral membrane protein on human monocytes (De Maria et al., 1994), or ligation of CD-23 molecule, a low affinity receptor for IgE expressed on the activated human monocytes (Dugas et al, 1995), have been shown to induce expression of iNOS and production of NO. It has been further shown that freshly isolated human peripheral blood monocytes do not express CD-23 molecule, but such an expression could be induced by treatment with IL-4. Although the mechanism of induction of NO production by human monocyte/macrophages may be different from that reported for murine macrophages, experimental studies have demonstrated the potential role of NO in the elimination of intra-cellular pathogens in human monocytes (Vouldoukis et al., 1995).

Mechanism of Action of NO

The cytotoxic effects of NO is primarily due to inactivation of enzyme involved in critical metabolic pathways in the target cells (James, 1995). Through the formation of iron-dinitrosyl-dithiolate complexes, NO inactivates several key metabolic enzymes with prosthetic groups (4Fe-4S) at their catalytic sites (Salerno, 1996). Nitrosylation of Fe-S centers is associated with inactivation of mitochondrial enzymes. NO also inactivates ribonucleotide reductase involved in DNA synthesis and cell proliferation and can also react with superoxide anions to form peroxynitrite (Beckman, 1996). Since the half life of NO is very short, a few seconds only, it is believed that its effects are limited to targets located very close to the NO source and, therefore, toxicity to surrounding tissues is expected to be minimal. However, it has also been reported that NO produced by activated macrophages binds to albumin and circulates as S-nitroso adduct of serum albumin and exerts cytotoxic effects on extracellular microorganisms (Stemler et al., 1992). S-nitroso-albumin therefore may represent a possible effector molecule of activated macrophages which can act at long distances.

Effector Functions of NO

Activated macrophages have the ability to recognize and eliminate tumor cells by various mechanisms which may require cell to cell contact or release to cytotoxic effector molecules. NO is now believed to be one of the effector molecules produced by macrophages which can induce apoptosis in tumor cells (Stuehr and Nathan, 1989; Cui et al., 1994). Interestingly, it has been shown that conversion of L-arginine into citrulline and NO corresponds to anti-tumor effects, whereas generation of ornithine and urea promotes tumor growth (Mills et al., 1992). On the other hand, tumor cells have been found to produce factors that downregulate the production of NO (Ding et al., 1990). Methods for upregulation of NO production by macrophages therefore hold promise for therapeutic effect against NO sensitive tumors.

Effector role of NO for intracellular killing of parasites has been extensively studied and there appears to be a general consensus that enhancement of NO production may have therapeutic effect against intracellular infections. Experimental studies on Leishmaniasis have shown that resistance to Leishmania infection is dependent on Th-1 directed cell mediated immune mechanisms and that susceptible mice strains can be protected against Leishmania infection by transfer of. Th-1 cells or by inducing Th-1 (IFN-γ) response in these animals (Sher and Coffman, 1992). It has also been shown that IFN-γ induced production of nitric oxide by macrophages could enhance intracellular killing of Leishmania parasite and that treatment of Leishmania infected mice with the NOS inhibtor

NMMA results in increased parasitic load (Green et al., 1990; Leiw et al., 1990). Recent demonstration that the macrophages derived from mutant mice lacking iNOS gene fail to produce NO after stimulation with IFN-γ plus LPS and also fail to control Leishmania infection provides conclusive evidence for effector role of NO (Wei et al., 1995).

Similarly the ability of Mycobacteria to grow within the macrophages is dependent on production of NO by infected macrophages (Denis, 1991; Chan et al., 1992). Treatment of macrophages with arginase before infection has been found to abrogate IFN-γ induced killing of intracellular Mycobacteria within murine macrophages (Denis, 1991). This is further confirmed by the experimental observation that administration of iNOS inhibitors exacerbate the infection (Chan et al., 1992). NO has also been shown to have anti-viral effects against herpes simplex (Croen 1993) and murine retroviruses (Akarid et al., 1995).

Even in non-macrophage-tropic parasitic infections like the intra-hepatic stages of malaria, NO has been shown to be an important effector molecule. Hepatocytes are capable of producing NO following activation by cytokines and bacterial products. In fact, IFN-γ, TNF-α and IL-6 have been reported to be involved in the NO induced killing of intrahepatic malaria parasites (Nussler et al., 1991). IFN-γ acts synergistically with other cytokines and plays a central role in NO formation in hepatocytes and inhibits development of intra-hepatic stages of Plasmodium (Mellouk et al., 1994). Bacterial products such as LPS, which induce formation of NO by hepatocytes, inhibit the development of intra-hepatic Plasmodium parasites in vitro and in vivo and this inhibitory effect is abrogated following simultaneous incubation with NOS inhibitor. There are also reports showing that production of high amounts of NO by splenic cells correlates with resistance to blood stages of malaria (Jacobs et al., 1995).

Plant Derived NO Inducers as Potential Therapeutic Agents

In view of the current understanding of the therapeutic potential of NO against a wide variety of infections and tumors, we are evaluating the plant materials for their ability to induce NO production by macrophages. The screening protocol includes measurement of NO production by murine peritoneal macrophages in response to bacterial LPS. Based on this screening procedure, a number of plant materials that are used in the Indian traditional medicine were subjected to activity guided solvent fractionation and chromatographic separation to identify, purify and characterize the active components. Two such compounds a glycoside (NII-78) and a glycoprotein (NII-70) which retained the biological activity were then tested for their therapeutic efficacy using the following animal models:

NO-Sensitive P-815 Tumor Implants in DBA/2J Mice

A murine tumor cell line (P815) sensitive to NO mediated killing was used to evaluate the therapeutic potential of the plant compound. Treatment with these compounds induced regression of subcutaneous P815 tumor implants in DBA/2J mice. The adoptive transfer of macrophages from treated animals to tumor bearing mice also induced tumor regression confirming the macrophage mediated therapeutic effect of NII compounds.

Leishmania Susceptible BALB/c Mice

BALB/c mice infected with *Leishmania major* through the hind footpad were treated with NII compounds, daily for 3–4 weeks. The treatment significantly reduced footpad lesion and inflammation. Treatment of *Leishmania donovani* infected Hamsters with these compounds also showed significant lowering of parasitic load in the spleens. Peritoneal macrophages isolated from Balb/c mice pre-treated with NII compounds for 3 days showed significant increase in production of NO in response to LPS. These macrophages also showed enhanced intra-cellular clearance of Leishmania parasites, ex vivo; this effect was abrogated when NO synthase inhibitor, NGMML-A, was added to the culture indicating that the intra-cellular clearance of the Leishmania was mediated by production of NO. These compounds, however, did not show any direct anti-leishmanial effect.

Opportunistic Infection in Tumor-Bearing Immunocompromised Mice

To evaluate the therapeutic efficacy of plant derived NO inducers against opportunistic infections, tumor (P-815) bearing DBA/2J mice were infected with *Micobacterium smegmatis*. This Mycobacterial species is a non-pathogenic strain and normal mice are able to eliminate the infection. However, we found that P-815 tumor bearing mice show progressive decline in their ability to produce nitric oxide and become susceptible to this infection. We therefore used this model to evaluate if NII compounds could restore immunocompetance and reduce parasitic load. Our results indeed showed that treatment with NII compounds could restore NO production by tumor bearing mice and also reduce the parasitic load in various organs.

While further studies on these plant compounds are in progress, our experimental data indicate that modulation of NO production by macrophages using plant derived immunomodulators could provide a cost effective and less toxic alternative to chemotherapy against tumor and infections or such molecules can be used in conjuction with anti-tumor or anti-biotic drugs for a synergistic action.

References

Akarid K., Sinet M. and Desforges B. Gougerot-Pocidalo M.A. (1995) J. Virol., **69**: 7001–7005.

Beckman, J.S. (1996) In: Nitric Oxide: principles and action (Lancaster J., Ed) Academic Press, New York, pp 1–82.

Croen, K.D. (1993) J. Clin. Invest. **91**: 2446–2452.

Cui, S., Reichner, J.R., Mateo, R.B., Albina, J.E. (1994) Cancer Res., **54**: 2462–2467.

De Maria, R., Cifone, M.G. and Trotta, R. (1994) J. Exp. Med. **180**: 1999–2004.

Ding, A., Nathan, C.F., Graycar, J., Deryneck, R., Stuehr, D.J. and Srimal, S. (1990) J. Immunol. **145**: 940.

Drapier, J.C., Wietzerbin, J. and Hibbs, J.B. (1988) Eur. J. Immunol., **18**: 1587–1592.

Dugas, B., Mossalayi, M.D., Damais, C. and Kolb, J.P. (1995) Immunology Today, **16**: 574–579.

Green, S.J., Meltzer, M.S., Hibbs, J.B. and Nacy, C.A. (1990) J. Immunol., **144**: 278–428.

Hibbs, J.B., Taintor, R.R. and Vavrin, Z. (1987a) Science, **235**: 473–476.

Hibbs, J.B., Vavrin, Z. and Taintor, R.R., (1987b) J. Immunol., **138**: 550–565.

Jacobs, P., Radzioch, D. and Stevenson, M. (1995), J. Immunol., **155**: 5306–5313.

James, S.L. (1995) Microbiol. Rev., **59**: 533–547.

Knowles, R.G. and Moncada, S. (1994) Biochem. J., **298**: 249–258.

Liew, F.Y., Millot, S., parkinson, C., Palmer, R.M.J. and Moncada, S. (1990), J. Immunol., **144**: 4794–4797.

Marletta, M.A. (1994) Cell, **78**: 927–930.

Mellouk, S., Hoffman, S.L. and Liu, Z.Z. et al. (1994) Infect. Immun. **62**: 4043.

Mills, C.D., Shearer, J., Evans, R. and Caldwel, M.D. (1992) J. Immunol. **149**: 2709–2714.

Modolell, M., Corraliza, I.M., Link, F., Soler, G. and Eichmann, K. (1995) Eur. J. Immunol., **25**: 1101–1104.

Moncada, S. and Higgs, E.A. (1995) FASEB, J., **9**: 1319–1330.

Nathan, C.F. and Hibbs, J.B. (1991) Curr. Opinion Immunol., **3**: 65–70.

Nussler, A.K., Drapier, C., Renia, L., Pied, S., Miltgen, F., Gentilini, M. and Mazier, D. (1991) Eur. J. Immunol., **21**: 227–230.

Salerno, J.C. (1996) In: Nitric Oxide: principles and action (Lancaster, J., Ed) Academic Press, New York, pp 83–110.

Sher, A. and Coffman, R.L. (1992) Ann. Rev. Immunol. **10**: 385–409.

Stemler, J.S., Simon, D.I., Jaraki, J.A., Osborne, Simon, D.I., Keaney, J., Vita, J., Singel, D., Valeri, C.R. and Loscalzo, J. (1992) Proc. Natl. Acad. Sci., USA, **89**: 7674.

Stuehr, D.J. and Nathan, C.F. (1989) J. Exp. Med., **169**: 1543.

Vouldoukis, I., Rivero-Moreno, V., Dugas, B., Quaaz, F., Becherel, P., Debre, P., Moncada, S. and Mossalayi, D.J. (1995) Proc. Natl. Acad. Sci., USA, **92**: 7804–7808.

Wei, X., Charles, I.G., Smith, A., Ure, J., Feng, G., Huang, F., Xu, D., Muller, W., Moncada, S. and Liew, F.Y. (1995) Nature, **375**: 408–411.